The Code for Empowered Healing

For Ourselves
& Our Planet

SG Williams
BSc.(Hons) RAc.

Copyright © 2023 Heart's Discovery

All rights reserved.

ISBN: 978-1-7775584-5-1

DEDICATION

This is for the light-workers, healers, star-seeds, enlightened beings and extraordinary humans, who have been showing us the way to a higher collective consciousness. It is in this state of being that we all come into our own power, to help ourselves, heal each other and change the future of our planet for the better. We all have an important voice to share by staying strong to what we know is true. This book is for you blessed seekers. May you discover your heart's desire.

CONTENTS

	Acknowledgements	i
1	Introduction	Pg# 9
2	Vibration, Frequency & Qi	Pg# 13
3	The Foundation	Pg# 21
4	Body - Qi	Pg# 37
5	Mind - Energy	Pg# 51
6	Spirit - Soul	Pg# 65
7	Healing Methods	Pg# 77
8	The Code	Pg# 105
9	Mastery & Transference	Pg# 113
	About the Author	Pg# 129

ACKNOWLEDGMENTS

I am thankful for my husband who sees me as I am and who first fell in love with my spirit. He has been a source of strength, encouraging me to act on my convictions. I also appreciate the many kind friends and clients, who have gifted me with much love, respect and insight. In particular Donna and Chris, your light will never be forgotten.

1 Introduction

Do not let the memories of your past limit the potential of your future. There are no limits to what you can achieve on your journey through life, except in your mind... Believe in your infinite potential...
 −   Roy T. Bennett, The Light in the Heart

Healing is not always a special calling. It comes naturally as we learn to see ourselves as something more, connected to everyone and everything. Healing is the result of caring about others and our planet. The process is a journey of self discovery to becoming whole and recognizing the goodness within oneself. The Code to Empowered Healing is the condensation of decades of research and experience, as a scientist and a healer. The Code was created as a blueprint to help others begin their own healing adventures.

Every cell in our bodies uses and gives off energy, at every level, from our complex brains to our simple individual cells. This energy vibrates in and around us in waveforms with amplitude (height) and frequency (number of waves in a time period). This energy is a form of communication and in the natural state, fuels healthy processes. There are repeatable steps and activities we can follow to raise personal vibration that can impact others in a positive way. The quality and quantity of energy is the key to healing.

However, to tap into the ability to heal one's self, others and the world, requires that we build Qi, raise Energy and connect to our Source on a solid foundation of wellness. Key techniques can be used at levels of the Body, Mind and Spirit to become more proficient. There are ways to access the power within us and magnify it, by connecting to the greater cosmic consciousness through mastery and transcendence.

Seeking such a path and being open to other realities, will increase the ability to affect beneficial change. Many seek a connection to all there is, a higher power, God or Spirit. Epiphanies from a oneness with nature, deep states of meditation, near death experiences, accidental brushes with death, mystical religious revelations, encounters with angels or other-worldly beings, or use of psychedelics, shamanic drumming and breath-work (as examples), can change us. The result is often a lasting profound sense of peace and love, in a place where time, death and fear do not exist.

The moment we experience an altered state of consciousness by accident or technique, our life paths often change. Generically speaking, these events signify that our core being-ness has connected with the collective and cosmic consciousness, that awakens us to the realization that we are something more. This can trigger a lifelong search for a way back to repeat that extraordinary moment in time. We are forever set on a path to enlightenment whether we want it or not. Healing is the natural by-product of this journey.

For those of us who intellectually know and have come to believe there is more to this world than what we are told, we hope for an encounter with the divine as proof. Then there are many of us who don't know what to believe, while others see musings about the spirit world, hogwash. Historically, the human race has always been ascribed to "the something more" philosophy. Our religions, myths, legends and stories are full of magic and other worldly beings and spirits. Think back to your early childhood when you still believed in the Tooth Fairy or could feel wonder and excitement in a cool bug or new flower. Over time, this sense of magic was discouraged and subdued by the expectation to grow-up.

We all affect the vibrations and collective consciousness in ways we do not see. Not everyone will find or seek an epiphany. However, recapturing the wonder of life will provide a fertile place to start on a path to wholeness. As more people wake up to their own personal power and realize who they really are, they can increase the positive healing energy in the collective consciousness. One cannot be connected to the higher power without feeling a profound love for self and others. This is just the kind of energy the world needs right now to balance out the uncertainty of current events. Therefore with a pure, grateful heart and clear intention, for yourself, others and the world, expect the best and it will happen. *The*

Code for Empowered Healing can help you do that.

2 FREQUENCY, VIBRATION & QI

If you want to find the secrets of the universe, think in terms of energy, frequency and vibration. - Nikola Tesla

Frequency and amplitude are properties of an energy wave form. Frequency is the number of waves in a period of time. Amplitude is the height of the vibrational wave. Generally speaking high frequency waves have taller and thinner sinusoidal waveforms, while those that rise and fall less often (lower frequency), have lower heights or amplitudes. Movement of the waves through space creates a vibration. Higher frequencies create greater amounts of vibration.

Everything is energy vibrating at particular frequencies. Solid objects have lower denser vibrations while invisible gasses have higher vibrations and more energy. There is no such thing as empty space. Just because we cannot see something, does not mean it is not there. We only see what is visible to us in a small range of the visible spectrum of light. There is so much of our world we cannot see, even though we know it is there through science.

The ethereal waves vibrating at high frequencies that we can't see, are often what we believe to be the source of life. In different cultures this energy in the body, that inhabits and animates everything, is known as Qi or chi, Prana, life force, spirit, consciousness, soul, Shen, soul-energy, universal life force, infinite spirit, higher power, omnipotent power, universal source, goddess, Tao, Brahman, God, Allah, god, holy spirit, universal consciousness, manitou, the light, vital force, vital principle, the creator, pneuma, etheric energy, odic force, mana, psychic power, the divine, all that is and the universal power of creation. These are the energy waves with frequency and amplitude that bind together everything in the universe.

Magnetism is a special kind of energy where groups of electrons in atoms spin in opposite directions, creating a measurable field. A physicist by the name of Cohen, in 1972, developed a method for detecting and measuring the natural magnetic fields produced by various organs of the human body. It was determined that every organ has a biomagnetic field that produces specific pulsating frequencies. He found that the brain had the strongest emissions. The Institute of Heart Math however has done extensive work demonstrating that the heart's electromagnetic field is much stronger than that of the brain and can be measured in feet radiating out from the body.

Electricity is energy created by the flow of electrons. Robert Becker, wrote a book called *The Body Electric*, where he mapped out the electrical resistance in the bodies of humans and other organisms. He found that our energetic anatomy closely resembles the same meridian pathways and acupuncture points, used in Traditional Chinese Medicine (TCM). He also determined that the strength and shape of our energetic signals could be weakened or made stronger by outside forces from the environment and that these signals are the key to healing. He also believed that the phenomenon of extra sensory perception (ESP) occurred through the transmission of low frequency waves and that electromagnetic pollution is a greater risk to our health that we initially realized.

The biofield is a measurable force in the body believed to be a combination of electromagnetic and life force energy. Many have determined that every aspect of who we are is reflected in our biofield frequencies. Heart-Math uses meditation and breathing techniques to create a coherence that activates the heart-brain relationship. It has been discovered that the heart sends more signals to the brain than vice versa. When a person achieves a harmonious link between the heart and the brain (resonance), the heart biofield becomes very large and leaps out from the person, affecting everyone around it. The mind's role in resonance with the heart means that our frequencies are not only affected by physical transmitters, but psychological changes.

This Heart-Mind relationship correlates well with TCM. Within our bodies the life force takes on particular characteristics and properties depending upon location and role. The Jing energy or Jing Qi, located in the kidneys, is our original essence and the life force we are born with. This is supplemented by the Gu Qi from our food and Qing Qi from the air we breathe. Together these produce our postnatal Qi. These combine in the chest to form our true or essential Zong Qi which is then transmuted to other forms for defence, immunity, organ systems, regulation of body functions and the creation and movement of Qi, blood and body fluids.

TCM also describes energy in the body, that is not Qi per say, but different kinds of Spirit energy. In TCM the same external world around us, is reflected in the internal micro-world of our bodies. Each organ system corresponds to the elements found in nature with specific roles in relationship with the other elements. Every element/organ system within our body has a spiritual energy associated with it. The Five Spirits in TCM are called the Five Shen. These spirits, residing in the Heart, Liver, Lungs, Spleen and Kidneys, are known as Shen, Hun, Po, Yi, and Zhi. Together they collectively form the greater overall Shen spirit or soul.

According to Giovanni Maciocia, Shen is one of the vital substances of the body. It is the most subtle and non-material type of Qi. Separately, the Shen of the heart alone is the energy responsible for the operation of the mind. Heart Shen regulates the activity of thinking, consciousness, self, insight, emotional life, memory, choices and will. However together the collective five-spirit Shen, can also be interpreted as consciousness, but is more aligned with soul-energy, God, psychic energy and the sacred, pertaining to heaven. The five-spirit Shen also means "to state", "to express", "to explain", "to stretch", "to extend". It is this aspect that reaches out to, or connects us to energy of the higher power and life force surrounding us. It allows us to project outwards, relate and communicate with others. This five-spirit Shen energy is what makes us human.

All living things are hardwired to detect energy as vibrational frequencies through mechanoreceptors in the skin, visible light frequencies through the eyes and sound wave frequencies through the ears. Energy vibrations are messages in the form of waves. These invisible signals trigger our many receptors and sensors and then travel through our nervous system pathways, to be processed by our brains. The ability to detect energy frequencies is an evolutionary feature to protect us.

All vibrational energy, even at low amplitudes, constantly feeds us signals, helpful and harmful, without our conscious knowledge. These messages have a profound effect on our physical body, our mental health and aging. Good vibes are oscillations that are smooth, even (sinusoidal) and mimic frequencies found in nature. Such vibrations flowing in an uninterrupted continuous manner, at natural frequencies, show up in our body as freedom from pain, proper functioning organs and a positive outlook on life. Harmful energy vibrations are choppy, uneven, non-synchronous and not harmonious with frequencies found in nature. These corrupted, sometimes weakened, or lowered frequencies can stagnate the flow of energy creating feelings of sluggishness, disease, pain and sadness or depression.

Regenerative Medicine is an area of medicine based in energy and vibrational science. Humans are not like machines and scientists recognize that there is a force that "animates" us and when that is gone, we disintegrate. They want to harness this life force to bring back the homeostasis of the body for healing. Even diseases have frequencies. Those vibrations are often choppy, non-synchronous and can be treated with good vibrations to counter and cancel diseased frequencies. Currently vibration is being used for reducing pain, healing wounds, increasing mobility, reducing inflammation, improving immunity and specific diseases such as Fibromyalgia and Parkinson's.

According to Dr. Royal R. Rife, every disease has a frequency. He found that certain frequencies can prevent the development of disease and that others would destroy disease. Substances with higher frequency will destroy diseases of a lower frequency. The study of frequencies raises an important question, concerning the frequencies of substances we eat, breathe and absorb. Many pollutants lower healthy frequency. Processed/canned food has a frequency of zero. Fresh produce has up to 15 Hz, dried herbs from 12 to 22 Hz and fresh herbs from 20 to 27 Hz.
– Susan Anderson

Visible light produces energy frequencies in a small range that we can see. Photomultipliers, extremely sensitive phototubes, can detect light that we can't see, in the ultraviolet and near infrared ranges at levels as small as an individual photon. With this, ultra weak light particles have been measured emerging from the hands and forehead. In fact all living organisms produce a continuous auto-luminescence (glow). Some researchers are using this signal to determine the progression of disease or aging, as damage to the body weakens our energy emissions. There are many things we can do to improve our health, boost our energy and increase our radiance by surrounding ourselves with high energy healthy options and practices.

When people are healing others, there are changes in the energy frequencies. Dr. Moga did studies on healing practitioners and was able to measure shifts in the emission of the magnetic fields of the practitioners while they performed healing treatments on others. She measured electromagnetic forces emitting the strongest from the heart, that could be detected several feet from the body. Shifts of 8-10 Hz were noted as healers invoked a compassionate presence that was shown to actively engage their bioenergetic field.

"Your personal vibration or energy state is a blend of the contracted or expanded frequencies of your body, emotions and thoughts at any moment. The more you allow your soul to shine through you, the higher your personal vibration will be."
– Penney Price

The secret to empowered healing lies in

understanding energy, vibration and frequencies and their impact on the body, mind and spirit. Being able to optimize various forms of energy, then direct it to a specific purposeful intention, fuelled by compassion, is a powerful healing tool. Cultivating emotions of compassion, empathy and gratitude, for example, will positively affect and increase personal healing power. This kind of active engagement of one's own bioenergetic field, produces a compassionate presence. When infused with wisdom, the healer can influence good energetic patterns in biofields to restore health, for self and others.

3 The Foundation

The foundation is the presence of a baseline fundamental overall wellness. In order to increase the capacity for healing, we need to treat ourselves as an important instrument in need of care and loving adjustments. This does not just include getting enough rest, eating nutritious foods and keeping the body fit. Getting in touch with nature helps us synchronize with our environment, so we can become more balanced. The world inside our bodies is a mirror of the world around us. Therefore we need to examine what we eat, how we eat, how we move and fine tune our lifestyles to become more aligned with the seasons. We also need to consider our internal state and intimate spaces as well as the external environment and the culture that envelopes us.

What and How we Eat

All foods should provide us with minerals, vitamins, protein, carbohydrates, fats and the water we need to build and transform for growth, maintenance, repair, immunity and metabolism for heat and energy. Minerals and vitamins are found in all foods and are needed for our metabolic processes. Vegetables, grain and fruit are good sources and also provide fibre to aid digestion and elimination. Protein is necessary for building blood, muscle, producing hormones and for healing. Good fats, mostly plant based, are needed for brain health, provide energy and protect the organs. Carbohydrates are the body's main energy source and the preferred source of energy of the brain.

All these food categories are needed for us to function well, including fat. Diets that restrict any of these areas can put our bodies out of balance. Some like tree mushrooms, berries, cruciferous and leafy green vegetables, legumes, tomatoes, nuts, whole grains, olive oil, fish and fermented foods, are considered superfoods because of the quality, quantity and wide range of micro nutrients for healing. Animal meat, dairy and eggs are the only complete proteins with all the amino acids we need and the only natural source of vitamin B12 (cobalamin). The key to health is in the kind and variety of foods we eat. Variety is important. Make sure to eat as many food groups as possible. Mix up your diet with new choices and expand your tastes.

Some experts believe we are malnourished because of our modern diets. Science is now looking back at data and trends pointing to the importance of the traditional diet. A traditional diet includes: fermented foods like sauerkraut, kimchi, yogurt, kombucha, pickles, seaweed, organ meats, grass fed beef, free range eggs, cod liver oil, fish eggs, fish such as salmon or herring, lots of vegetables cooked with a little fat, cooked green vegetables, kale, broccoli, cauliflower, turnip, leeks, onion, mushrooms (especially those growing on trees like chaga), brightly coloured vegetables, soup stocks (especially bone broth), whole milk, butter, lard, bacon fat, coconut oil, pure olive oil and fruits in season like berries.

The food source is also key. The quality of the nutrients depends on the type of food, how it was procured and how fresh it is. Eat real, whole, fresh, natural food found as close to the source as possible (local). Learn about where it grows, how and when it is harvested, the use of pesticides and the contents of the soil. If we could eat right from our own yards, that would be best. In fact we can. Many of what people consider to be weeds are actually edible and good for you. Wild grown plants often have more beneficial components, due to the vigour and variation of their genetics, than our few homo-genetic and domesticated foods. Just be sure to do some research and understand the correct identification of what you eat before it is consumed. This is particularly important for wild harvested mushrooms and other fungi.

How food is cooked will determine the availability of essential nutrients and how much of that we can absorb. Over cooking may lose some of the quality of components, while raw foods make it difficult for us to absorb the nutrients. In TCM (traditional Chinese medicine) foods have five properties of energy (cold, cool, neutral, warm, hot) and five flavours (bitter, sweet, pungent, salty, sour). These properties all have different effects on the movement of energy in the body and correlate to the function of specific organs. These properties are affected by the way the food is prepared.

Overly pungent (spicy) food for example, or dry food can aggravate the stomach causing heat or yin deficiency problems. Cold or raw foods can cause stagnation with bloating, gas, flatulence or pain. If you already have a cold imbalance, then it is OK to eat spicy foods. If you already have a heat imbalance, then cold and raw is OK. The situation is different for every person. If you find you are ravenous for food at certain times of the day, chances are you have stomach heat. Food consisting of a warm, moist, neutral balance is best.

How much we eat is important too. Being overweight can affect our health. Research on mice found that those on a calorie reduced diet, tended to live longer. In the same way many claim that fasting is good for our longevity. However, people who were too thin, have also been found to have a reduced longevity. Therefore it is all about balance, eating in moderation and resourcing a wide variety of foods to make sure we get all the nutrients we need.

When you eat, how you eat, your frame of mind and the regularity of meals, also affects nutritional intake and ultimate wellness. It is important to chew well and eat meals at regular times. The peak time for the stomach to digest is between 7am and 9am and it is best to eat meals at the same time every day. Don't eat too fast, nibble, read while eating, eat too late at night, think about work, worry, or be sad or angry while eating. Emotional strain is a detriment to good digestion. A positive frame of mind is important. Worrying, over thinking and over analyzing, even when not eating, can affect the ability to absorb nutrients. Over a long period of time, emotional upset while eating, can lead to chronic deficiencies and malnutrition.

Our food should be our medicine. This means not just eating what tastes good, but developing a mindset to eat what our body needs. Often cravings are a signal that there is something lacking in our diet. Learning to pay attention and sense our body's reactions to foods, will help us differentiate binge eating that leads to little satisfaction, versus a credible craving for something we need. The latter feels very satisfying to the body and the desire for that item will end after eating. We should be eating to give our body what is needed and using our everyday meals as medicine by paying attention to the signals our body is using to communicate with us.

Everything we need to be healthy and all the tools we need to care for ourselves, should be readily available in nature. Traditional medicine practitioners use dandelion as a tonic in spring, coltsfoot for the lungs, plantain leaves to stop bleeding and chamomile for sleep. While some plant compounds form the basis for western pharmaceuticals, the wisdom of plant medicine has been missed. Some cultures and Western herbalists have well developed effective herbs and formulas that have been used for thousands of years, that are well balanced, gentle and safe. Most require a qualified practitioner and a correct diagnosis before prescribing. There are however formulas that a lay person can use in moderation, by purchasing over the counter.

It doesn't make sense that humankind would come into existence without all the accessible tools needed for health and survival. If the birds and little creatures in this world have everything they need to thrive, why not us? Many cultures use herbs for health and healing. In Europe, it is common to see wall-to-wall shelves of dried herbs, along with rows of bottles, pills and supplements. Therefore our food and the natural inhabitants we find in our immediate surroundings, can and should be used as medicine, to correct health problems and put us back in balance.

I believe that for every illness or ailment known to man, that God has a plant out here that will heal it. We just need to keep discovering the properties for natural healing. - Vannoy Gentles Fite

How we Move

If you don't move, you will lose muscle mass, put on weight and lack energy. The Qi in the body needs to flow. When it is not flowing properly, the result is pain, dysfunction and symptoms of imbalance. In order for it to flow there needs to be enough fluid, blood and yin that is acquired by living properly and eating right.

Lack of movement can cause all kinds of obstructions like cold and damp conditions that can cause the clear rivers of Qi to behave more like muddy puddles. When there is no movement of Qi, there are deficiencies that can cause fatigue and failure to transform and transmute fluids properly. This can cause weight gain, digestive issues, water retention, swelling and more.

Unless you are trying to increase endurance or strength for a particular purpose, you don't need to run a marathon or work out in the gym. Walking at a good pace, in the fresh air, is perfect. Ideally you want to do at least twenty or thirty minutes a day. Wear comfortable shoes and if you can walk in nature, looking at the trees. Breathing in the oxygen the trees put out, has the extra benefit of helping you feel calmer and more grounded.

There are many forms of exercise that a person could take up. Swimming, jogging, biking, yoga, on a team, or as an individual sport, are all good, as long as it is regular and does not cause injuries. Qigong is an ancient Chinese form of therapeutic movement that is similar to Tai Chi, but concentrates on the medical aspects of health and supporting body systems. "Qi" stands for the Qi energy that is being cultivated and "Gong" means mastery. It is beautifully gentle, employs breathing techniques, visualization and is designed to keep meridian channels open for improved immunity, focus and balance.

Qi(chi) is the Chinese term for life energy, or life spirit, a vital force that flows through all living things. It is an essential part of Traditional Chinese Medicine, acupuncture, Qigong and the Chinese martial arts. When our Qi is in harmony, we tend towards wellness, health and longevity. When our Qi is in disharmony we tend towards disease, suffering and collapse. - Subtle Energy Sciences

...

When you cultivate balance and harmony within yourself, or in the world, that is Tai Chi. When you work and play with the essence of energy of life, nature and the universe for healing, clarity and inner peace, this is Qigong. - Roger Jahnke

Lifestyle and the Seasons

The ancient sages tell us to live in harmony with nature and the patterns of the seasons. Spring is the time of the wood element. This element represents the liver and gallbladder. If it is well balanced, you will feel supple, resilient and be able to move and bend easily both physically and emotionally. You will have clear plans, know what you want to accomplish and why. You will have energy, willpower and the information to make good decisions. If not in balance, you may have red, itchy or watery eyes, stiff tendons, bizarre dreams and reproductive or menstrual issues. You may feel unmotivated, irritable or angry. Therefore rest, dress warm, protect yourself from draft or wind and avoid cold salads, cool drinks and fast cooked foods. Nourish yourself with immune boosting herbs (astragalus for example) and eat slow cooked soups (with warming herbs such as ginger and garlic) and stews (with antivirals like rosemary, sage or thyme).

Summer is the time of the fire element and is about the heart, relationships, joy, laughter and heat. This can translate to passion and a focus on intimate relationships and socializing. If in balance, the heart helps us be our intuitive true self and the small intestine will give us good clarity, discernment and judgment. These, in balance, produce good Shen that can be seen in eyes that are bright, clear and present. If out of balance, a person does not want to talk, socialize, has mood swings, dream disturbed sleep or possible heart palpitations. If so, drink lots of fluids, eat meals that are lightly cooked, steamed or simmering with high heat, short cooking times, bitter foods like dandelion as well as Swiss chard, romaine, broccoli, celery, alfalfa, apples, cucumber and watermelon.

Late summer is a time of peace and of abundance. The organs of this earth element, the spleen and stomach, roots us, transforms and transports our food to nourish us. In balance, we are sensitive and reactive to the needs of others. If not, we become overly worried, obsessive, filled with self-doubt and selfishly turn inward. Physically we have digestive issues, bloating, lack of energy and may experience more bruising. It is best to ease up on mental stress and overthinking and avoid foods high in fats or sugar. Instead, focus on a regular eating schedule with warming, neutral foods that are cooked and easy to digest. Qi boosting herbs like ginseng are also helpful.

Fall-autumn is the metal element represented by the lungs and large intestine. These govern the defensive Wei Qi, skin, nose, water passages, mucous membranes, respiration, the strength of our voice and the emotion of grief. This season can bring more lung issues and lowered immunity if we become pensive, worried or sad. Eat pungent, savoury, spicy and warming foods, nutritious soups, stews and herbs to boost immunity. Don socks and scarves to keep you warm and stay positive. It helps to be grateful for everything no matter how small.

Winter is the time for contemplation, introspection, hibernating, conserving energy and going inward. This water element is represented by the kidneys, bladder. These influence hearing, the bones, hair growth, fertility, the emotion of fear as well as willpower, hope and potential. The Ming Men, between the kidneys, store our life force called Jing. Winter is the most important time to slow down and regenerate. Avoid strenuous exercise, fasting and cleansing diets. Salty and bitter flavours such as miso, seaweed and soya sauce combined with bitter turnip, warming black pepper, cinnamon, onion and protein like egg, black bean and pork, slow cooked at low temperature, are ideal. Especially beneficial is any soup made with bone broth.

Intimate Spaces and Support Systems

Living things create good vibrant energy and life force and it is important to feel good about our homes, offices and places of work. When these places work well and inspire us, that affects our well-being. When our intimate spaces get cluttered and messy, the energy stagnates and affects how we feel. When we bring in fresh air, lots of light and pay attention to the layout, design and geographical features, good Qi can enter, linger and flow abundantly.

Feng Shui is an ancient practice of positioning homes and designing structures, to ensure good fortune and the proper flow of Qi. A house with land sloping upward behind it and sloping downwards in the front is good. Lush vegetation and water in the front would be ideal but there are many ways to improve Qi in whatever setting you have. Getting rid of clutter is the first fix. The rest can be done with proper placement of furniture, accessories and colours.

Each area of the house has unique qualities and is believed to affect specific areas of your life. The centre of the house represents the Earth element and mainly correlates to health, well-being, integrity, sympathy, self-care and the intellect. This space should be clean, vibrant, healthy and grounded. Living green plants, with rounded, not sharp leaves, stone or pottery accents and colours with yellows, browns and beige earth tones are good. Some recommend pictures of the earth, stars, sunrise, vegetables or fruit to enhance the energy here.

The other eight areas depend on what school of Feng Shui you adopt. Using the compass method, the north corner of the house, room or property, represents water, career success, wisdom, kidney and bone health. The Qi of this area is enhanced by a water feature or the colours dark blue or black. The south corner represents the Fire element, fame, reputation, prosperity, joy, heart health and is improved by the positioning of a light source (tall lamp or candle) and red, orange or yellow accents.

The east represents the Wood element, wind, thunder and influences family dynamics. Green colours and wood items enhance the Qi in this area and it is a good place to put happy pictures of family members. The west and Metal element is about creativity, children, self-worth, helpful people, spirits, authority and respect. Metal objects and the colours gold, silver and white benefit this area. The west is a good place for children's artwork or pictures of people who have helped or inspired you.

Other design features you need to watch for are areas of clutter, sharp corners, ceiling beams or low sloping ceilings. These features can negatively affect the Qi by causing it to stagnate, become too sharp or oppressive. Steep stairs and long hallways can cause the Qi energy to speed up. These deterrents can be improved through proper placement of furniture, plants, mirrors, crystals and wind chimes to dissipate, slow down or redirect the energy path. Furniture should be spaced so there is a good flow without blocking movement or sight lines. However the most important feature is being able to enjoy your living and work space while keeping it functional and practical.

Beyond Feng Shui, the physical design and geographical aspects of our home, it is what makes a house, a home, that is important. For most of us, home is our haven and safe place. It is where we are nourished and protected, where we and our loved ones grow and interact in a healthy way. This is where we can host our friends and extended families so they can benefit from the good Qi we have cultivated. Keeping the relationship aspects of our home in good order, affects the physical well-being for all the stakeholders and those who visit. This means taking care and maintaining the relationships that inspire us and distancing ourselves from those people that have a negative impact on us.

The Environment, Society and Culture

The external environment can affect our well-being in more ways than just the absence of toxicity, clean food, water and air. Our genes also play a large role. Signals from our behaviour and the environment, from outside our genetic code (Epigenetics), impacts the RNA and the production of cells. Therefore our external environment can change gene expression and how our bodies grow, change and adapt. According to the Ottawa Charter for Health Promotion:

The fundamental conditions and resources for health are peace, shelter, education, food, income, a stable ecosystem, sustainable resources, social justice and equity. Improvement in health requires a secure foundation in these basic prerequisites.

Science has shown that everything is connected even though the medical profession has yet to acknowledge it. Illness, therefore, is a process involving a combination of mental, emotional as well as physical, variables. Some have acknowledged this and even believe that all trauma in our life, has an impact on our physical health, depending upon how we internalize those events. From before birth, until the day we die, we must deal with tragedy. Those who find themselves loved by parents and families with caring supportive relationships, will fare better than most.

Our cultural attitudes of racism, sexism, educational and mobility barriers for the elderly and disabled, our wage systems, costs of housing and rent, the cost of food, bullying, injustice and the state of our justice and policing systems, are also factors impacting our health and well-being. In addition, social media can harm one's self-worth when people believe that status, wealth and popularity is important. Instead of being appreciated for who we are, these external artificial standards make people feel unworthy. Our world unfortunately is rife with hate disguised as judgment, bullying and gossip and is an epidemic in our communities and workplaces.

Hate causes us to harden our hearts, to shield us for protection. However, that wall also blocks delicate feelings of love, kindness and generosity. As people become disconnected from their vulnerable true selves, they become less human, more robotic, less caring, less empathetic and lose compassion. Many illnesses, addictions and crime are the natural consequences of an unnatural, non-healthy, hateful world. It causes people to lash out in anger, disrespect laws and norms and turn to self medication or detrimental lifestyles to deaden the pain.

A toxic society should never be accepted. Do not think because something is considered normal or expected, by most, that it is normal and OK. In order to heal we must protect ourselves from negative societal expectations. Introspection will help us find out why we do what we do and how to respond differently. Over time inner wisdom will uncover patterns and insight that can enlighten and liberate us towards wholeness. Opening our hearts to recover our empathy, will urge us towards compassion and the desire to make things better for others who are suffering.

"When we flee our vulnerability, we lose our full capacity for feeling emotion. We cannot selectively numb our feelings. When we build a wall to keep the pain out (or in), we also keep out the joy and peace of mind that are achievable." - Dr. Gabor Mate

...

For if medicine is really to accomplish its great task, it must intervene in political and social life. It must point out the hindrances that impede the normal social functioning of vital processes, and affect their removal – Rudolf Virchow (nineteenth century German physician)

In summary, the baseline foundation of wellness involves nutrition, how we move, the state of our intimate surroundings, personal support systems, the cleanliness of our external environment and the societal culture that surrounds us. It also means we need to pay attention, not just to our own bodies, families, homes and intimate spaces, but to the world around us and the fate of others. Suffering of others affects everyone. Living well and in alignment with the seasons, will provide the abundance of Qi, Energy and connection to Soul-Self, needed to fuel compassion to heal ourselves, others and our world.

The highest degree of a medicine is Love. - Paracelsus

4 Body - Qi

The foundation described in the beginning of this book, provides us with a baseline of wellness. Now that we understand more about the nature of energy in and surrounding us, we can go beyond the basics. We can increase and fine-tune the Qi of our body, using specific practices and techniques.

Bathe your Body in Good Qi

Just think about how good it feels to walk in the forest, along the beach and stand in the sun on a clear day. Sitting in the sun every day, just for a few moments, can alleviate depression. Everyone loves to be next to the water and walk along the beach. Water holds and concentrates Qi energy and we feel rejuvenated just by looking out the window at the trees and the water. This is nature increasing the vibration of our personal energy and healing us.

In traditional Chinese medicine (TCM) the Qi

flows into our bodies and circulates through it. When this life-force is stagnant or when blockages occur, patterns of dysfunction occur in our bodily functions and our emotions. When there is no flow, there is pain. Acupuncture based in TCM, is specifically designed to diagnose the root causes of energy imbalances and treat them. Energy healing therapies like Therapeutic Touch® and Reiki, also focus on opening up this flow of energy, so the frequencies are harmonious. Talk therapy used by psychologists, helps by removing emotional and mental blockages impacting how we relate to ourselves and those around us. Getting rid of blockages on all levels, heals our bodies.

The only way to extend our lives is to supplement the Qi we were born with through the air we breathe and the food we eat. We conserve the life force we were born with, by the way we live. Being in nature supplies high energy directly to our lungs especially when the air is clean. I believe salt air has a higher vibration because as a food, good natural salt has lots of minerals and is considered a high energy food.

Eating a traditional diet focused on natural, not processed, whole not modified, as well as fresh and local, ensures a good vibration in the food we eat. High energy foods are fresh and natural fruit, herbs, vegetables, spices, nuts and oils. Plants in particular have spent their lives converting the sun's rays, the air and the minerals of the earth from nothing into something pretty spectacular.

Our food choices, sources and preparation carries particular frequencies. Higher energy foods include those that have not been processed, tainted with chemicals, modified or changed. The highest frequency foods are said to be fresh leafy vegetables, fruits and fresh eggs for example. Cooked foods have lower frequencies but this must be weighed against the ability to absorb nutrients. Raw foods and whole grains, while being more alive, are harder to digest, so steaming, sprouting and fermenting helps get more value from them. Buying local and often can have a positive effect on the resulting quality of the foods.

Being in tune with your body and the messages it is sending you helps you to adjust to a healthier lifestyle. One of the jobs as a holistic healer is the questioning at the beginning of each session. How was your sleep? Did you pee in the night, how many times? Were you awakened by dreams, what happened? Any pain, gas, burping after eating? What does your bowel movement look like? Any heart palpitations, hot flashes, unusual sweating, cough, shortness of breath, skin rashes? Do you have any pain, was it alleviated by pressure, by cold or by heat? We can all be our own detectives, investigating and interpreting our own body language. The more we pay attention to the body's messages and respond to them, the better we will be at alleviating the symptoms of disease before they become a problem. In fact we can prevent many diseases this way.

Cultivate and Gather Qi

Once we feed ourselves energy, it is important that we try to conserve and concentrate that acquired post heaven Qi. We can only digest well when we are happy, calm and thinking good thoughts. Qigong helps pull more energy from our surroundings. Then slow, deep breathing helps us make more efficient use of it. In this way we can maximize the food and air to give us the most nutrients.

You can use your hands or finger tips to tap on acupuncture points or whole meridians to raise the vibration of your body. You do not need needles for these points, although the needling is the most powerful way to use them. Points along your eyebrows and on your cheek bones or the top of your head can provide stimulation for the senses, open the orifices and "pull up" your Qi. The Emotional Freedom Technique (EFT) uses many of these points. Each area taps into meridians that relate to specific emotions. These sets of points can be used to calm the mind, reduce anxiety, fear and worry, increase confidence and improve the flow of energy, Qi and blood.

There are 12 primary meridians (energy pathways) in the body and 8 extraordinary pathways. Each travels along routes at 3 levels from near the surface to the deep interior. Half of the primary channels are yin and reach into the solid yin organs (Lung, Spleen, Heart, Kidney, Pericardium, Liver). The other half are yang and reach into the hollow yang organs (Large Intestine, Stomach, Small Intestine, Bladder, Gallbladder, Triple Warmer). Special points along the surface of the meridians, called acupuncture points, have different, unique actions on the body and activate many beneficial, functional, healing, anti-inflammatory, immune boosting, regulatory and balancing properties. They all activate the flow of energy in the channels. You can also use your fingers to locate, press and hold specific acupuncture points. This is called acupressure.

Build and Move the Qi

In addition to acupuncture points, movement like Qigong, is a great way to raise your vibration. Start by swinging the arms from front to back while hitting the area below the navel and lower back, repeatedly. This wakes up the core energy centre for the body. The Eight Brocade is a common set of Qigong movements that opens any blockages and gets the Qi flowing. It was developed in China and has been used routinely for thousands of years. It is easy to remember and easy to do while being extremely beneficial. At the end of the movements, rising on your toes and plunking yourself down on your heels, sends vibrations throughout the body for a final shake up.

Tap into Frequencies

Specific sounds have vibrations that can target particular areas of the body for healing. Drums, gongs, singing bowls, tuning forks, our voices and music tuned to nature, can be used for healing purposes. Music can evoke higher frequency emotions like love, empathy or compassion for example. Sound therapy is not only extremely enjoyable, but can push your choppy, wayward energy waves back into their natural, smooth and harmonic shape. Sounds with frequencies found in nature help us get our own vibrations back on track. Creating natural sounds or using a water fountain, can improve the indoor environment when you can't get outdoors.

With the tuning forks, the various "Ohm" vibrations of 68.05 or 138.1 Hertz (Hz) of can be used for relaxation. A 528 Hz fork is good for healing and very high pitched forks, in the 4000+Hz range, are believed to clear negative energy and connect to angelic realms. Tibetan singing bowls that tune to specific scales can resonate with the energy centres of the body (the chakras) to facilitate overall healing and well-being.

Drumming has been used all over the world by every indigenous culture, since ancient times. These pleasing vibrations are used for entertainment, cultural ceremonies. Shamans use specific beat frequencies, to achieve a meditative state that allows them to connect to the spirit world. Modern research has found that it is beneficial for the immune system, physical healing and the release of emotional trauma, grief, anxiety, depression and behavioural issues. Drum circles provide a powerful experience with patterns of beats that naturally emerge. You can feel the vibration of the circle, and the energy of everyone present, dramatically increase.

Studies have also shown that certain music is more effective for impacting our well-being than others, because of specific frequency blueprints. The current reference for tuning musical instruments is 440 Hz. However, music tuned at 432 Hz or using the Solfeggio scale, are tuned to natural vibrations. These frequencies on this ancient scale, first used in Gregorian Chants, are divisible by the numbers 3, 6 and 9 and are in tune with nature from a mathematical perspective. A number of music artists like Scott Huckabay, have chosen to create music by re-tuning their instruments to these natural frequencies. It has been found that naturally tuned music has produced remarkable results, on the ability to elevate our spirits.

If parts of the body become imbalanced, they may be healed through projecting the proper and correct frequencies back into the body. - Jonathan Goldman, Healing Sounds: The Power of Harmonics

Scents are transmitters of energy. Pure, all natural, essential oils, stimulate cell receptors in the nose, sending emotional responses through the limbic system. The oils must be distilled from plants found in nature, not scented or enhanced with man-made chemicals. Pure oils from natural sources are therapeutic and activate the olfactory system (sense of smell) to trigger the brain and affect mechanisms for mood or healing. These scents can move us, bring back memories, improve memory, give us courage, change our mood and help us feel more positive, energized, happy, relaxed, aroused, sleepy or creative.

The vibrations from pure essential oils can be used indoors for healing. Lavender oil has a wide range of benefits including muscle relaxation and antimicrobial properties. Frankincense has been used for centuries for anti-aging. Bergamot is a great choice for depression, anxiety and nervous tension while lavender is better at calming and balancing emotional extremes. Neroli, from the orange blossom, and roman chamomile are very relaxing and can help with sleep. The former also inspires confidence and is an aphrodisiac. Oil from orange leaves or the fruit peel, is calming, sedating and enhances the feeling of optimism.

To increase mental stamina and improve concentration, add basil or black pepper. To help feel more grounded, less irritable or anxious, add fir, black spruce or marjoram. Fir and black spruce also help with respiratory issues. Marjoram can be sedating and also eases joint pain. Rosemary oil is also used for mental focus and pain. Niaouli, from the same family as Tea Tree, is great as a decongestant when you have a cold or flu, while Tea Tree oil is used largely for skin conditions.

To improve your outlook on the world, some of the oils can do this by balancing the emotions in addition to relieving stress. Cardamom and oranges remind us of life's abundance and combat negative thinking. Lemon, clary sage, grapefruit, tangerine and jasmine are happy oils and are great revitalizers and stimulants. Elemi and spearmint are calming. Spikenard is very calming (sedating). Clary sage is good for panic attacks but has estrogenic action. Tangerine and grapefruit are also good to enhance weight loss.

... Science is now confirming... Essential oils have healing properties on both physical and emotional levels. Absorbed through the skin and via the olfactory-brain connection through inhalation, they have been considered among the most therapeutic

and rejuvenating of all botanical extracts throughout the ages. - Valerie Gennari Cooksley

Crystals are natural solids with well ordered and defined molecular structures. Each type of crystals forms a particular signature shape, in their original earthbound environment. These special and often extremely beautiful stones have distinct frequencies that are stable and uniform. Their energy resonates from the earth and produces vibrations that align with nature and the human body. Ancient people have been known to use various crystals such as lapis lazuli, carnelian, emerald, quartz and turquoise in ceremony and healing to affect energy, as far back as ancient Sumer, Mesopotamia and Egypt, 6,000 to 10,000 years ago.

Crystal energy was believed to have a positive effect on spiritual, emotional and physical healing. While there is not a lot of science to back up the claims of crystal healing as a medicine, many have claimed significant positive effects when using them for mental and emotional support. Crystals do have unique and interesting piezoelectric properties of producing electricity (AC alternating current) when under mechanical pressure, vibration and latent heat. Some crystals also have the ability to stabilize energy wave patterns. Quartz and tourmaline are often used in electronics because of this.

Frequencies emitted by crystals can also support us in various ways. Some wear crystals as amulets to increase clarity of thinking, positive emotion and personal power, for example. Citrine is often used to strengthen positive energy, healthy boundaries and personal power. Clear quartz and granite rocks speckled with quartz, can amplify the good vibrations of all other crystals and help maintain a connection with the higher self. Amethyst is exceptionally high in vibrational frequencies and is good at clearing rooms of negative energies. Its purple colour, corresponds to the crown chakra, that connects us to our intuition and is particularly good to have for healing rituals. In general, a stone that is right for you, can increase the feeling of being grounded, improve mood and can help with the feeling of being connected and at peace.

Every colour has an energy frequency. Chromotherapy is a practice that uses the vibrations of particular colours to move and influence organ systems that may be out of balance or diseased. In the Indian tradition, there are seven energy centres. Each has a location, frequency and a corresponding colour. The root chakra (at the base of the torso), vibrates with red, the sacrum with orange, the solar plexus with yellow, the heart with green, the throat with light blue, the third-eye (between the eyebrows), with indigo blue and the crown chakra (above the top of the head) with the colour purple.

Each chakra and colour also resonate with particular emotional and psychological themes. The Root chakra is the base of our sense of stability and security in the world. The Sacral chakra is our creative and sexual energy. The Solar Plexus chakra governs our willpower and self esteem. The Heart chakra is all about relationships and connecting to others. The Throat chakra defines our ability to communicate and the Third Eye chakra is our intuition. The Crown chakra represents our higher self and our connection to the divine. To balance or strengthen any of these areas, wearing the corresponding colour or viewing the colour through a tinted lens, can help improve that weakness. The key is to expose yourself to the frequencies that the colour emits, to augment or correct the frequencies of that energy centre.

Emotions also correlate to colour frequencies. We have always heard that "seeing red" means anger, "feeling blue" represents sadness, "yellow bellied" refers to cowardice, "green" is associated with envy and black with grief. These traditional sayings do have some bearing in science. According to studies, the hue, tint and brightness of colours not only represents emotions but has a physiological effect on how we feel. In general it has been proven that brighter more saturated colours evoke positive emotions. Negative feelings being associated with more muted hues.

All these techniques raise and smooth-out frequencies into waves with more energetic, healthy, sinusoidal waves. Eating well, spending time in nature, activating the meridians, listening to healing sounds, using pure scents, colours and crystals, are all methods and sources of good energy. Movement like Qigong not only helps us gather Qi but keeps the energy flowing properly. Everything around us is a symphony of frequencies in many forms.

The key to enjoying and benefiting from this concert of life, is to listen to the messages your body provides and find a way to be in resonance with yourself and the world around you. Each season has vibrational properties that naturally align with the macrocosm and within our own microcosms. These patterns of synchronicity and relationships have been studied for centuries by ancient physicians.

From the Maoshing Ni's version of the Yellow Emperor's Classic of Medicine (written 2000+ years ago):

In the past, people practised the Tao, the Way of Life. They understood the principle of balance, of yin and yang, as represented by the transformation of the energies of the universe. Thus, they formulated practices such as Dao-in, an exercise combining stretching, massaging, and breathing to promote energy flow, and meditation to help maintain and harmonize themselves with the universe. They ate a balanced diet at regular times, arose and retired at regular hours, avoided over-stressing their bodies and minds, and refrained from overindulgence of all kinds... thus it is not surprising that they lived over one hundred years...

...

...The accomplished ones of ancient times advised people to guard themselves against, zei feng, disease causing factors. On the mental level, one should remain calm and avoid excessive desires and fantasies, recognizing and maintaining the natural purity and clarity of the mind... Previously, people led a calm and honest existence, detached from undue desire and ambition; they lived with an untainted conscience and without fear. They were active but never depleted themselves. Because they lived simply, these individuals knew contentment... Since they were

happy with their position in life, they did not feel jealousy or greed. They had compassion for others and were helpful and honest, free from destructive habits. They remained unshakable and unswayed by temptations, and they were able to stay centred even when adversity arose. They treated others justly, regardless of their level of intelligence or social position...

...

...Not so long ago (the)... achieved beings, who had true virtue, understood the way of life, and were able to adapt and to harmonize with the universe and the seasons. They too were able to keep their mental energy through proper concentration... These achieved beings did not live like normal human beings, who tended to abuse themselves. They were able to travel freely to different times and places since they were not governed by conventional views of time and space. Their sense perceptions were super-normal, going far beyond the sight and hearing of ordinary human beings. They were also able to preserve their life spans and live in full health, much as the immortals did.

5 Mind - Energy

The foundation of mental wellness involves learning to accept who you are. At the first level we need to develop reasons to respect our journeys and free ourselves from self destructive behaviours. The next level of growth involves going beyond mental stability by becoming present and conscious to the operation of one's own mind as a tool. Only then, can we learn how to influence and improve it.

Emotions and the Mind

Good physical health requires us to pay attention to the signals our body provides, to help us adjust our lifestyles. Signs of imbalances may come in the form of physical ailments but often come in the form of emotion and mind chatter. We need to be open to exploring this by being present, practising introspection, learning, acquiring knowledge and challenging our beliefs through our experiences. Identifying and removing blockages, barriers, harmful habits, addictions and self destructive behaviours, may require professional help and supportive people. These foundational habits will open a gateway to introduce us to the nature of our subconscious, our soul-self, self-love and universal unconditional love, needed for empowered healing.

Emotional Intelligence (EQ) is a measure of the ability to manage our emotions in a way that produces beneficial behaviour and optimal choices in decision making. It consists of four abilities: identifying how others feel; using emotion to assist the thinking process; understanding the root cause of the emotion; and being able to manage the emotions.

Those with a high EQ know what they are feeling, have good emotional self-control, are able to think clearly when experiencing strong emotions. They are able to make decisions based on their hearts and not just their heads. This makes them better able to get in touch with their passions and find a path in life that is fulfilling.

Suppressing emotions makes it harder to find our life path. It can also make us sick. Our life force needs to be flowing appropriately for us to be healthy. Just as blockages in the flow of Qi from trauma can cause pain, extremes in emotions affect the flow of Qi causing Qi and blood stagnation, heat, dampness and phlegm. These patterns can produce a long list of physiological imbalances and physical symptoms. For example:

- Anger and guilt causes Liver Qi to rise creating symptoms such as headaches, high blood pressure, reproductive issues, vision loss and other issues such as depression and insomnia.

- Worry and pensiveness knots the Spleen Qi and Stomach Qi, resulting in possible digestive issues, weak muscles, fatigue, easy bruising, bleeding, varicose veins and other issues.

- Sadness and grief dissolves Lung Qi. This weakens the lungs and our immunity and can bring on respiratory issues, skin conditions and make us more vulnerable to colds and flu.

- Shock and fear causes Kidney Qi to descend and dissolve. This along with overwork can cause weakened fertility, bladder problems, hearing loss, per-mature grey hair, sore knees and back.

- All emotions slow down the Heart Qi which houses the mind (cognition) and the Shen (ruler of the Spirit). This may create anxiety and mood swings between happy, sad with insomnia.

If you find yourself feeling strong emotions, get in touch with what you are feeling. Don't get busy so you don't have to think about it. Don't blame someone else for feeling the way you do. Often we only see the shadow of the cause of our emotional imbalance when we see it reflected in someone else. Use the emotion as a fishing line to see what else may be swimming around in the depths of the unconscious. Only you can allow yourself to feel the way you do.

Also our health can affect our emotions. The physical, spiritual and mental aspects of our being are all connected. When you don't eat, get enough sleep or suffer from acute or chronic disease combined with the need to take drugs, these things can have an affect on our emotions.

Meditation

Meditation is an important tool for self discovery, exploration and training of voluntary control of thought. The benefits include the ability to achieve a state of calmness, the wisdom to see life events from an impassioned perspective and the differentiation of your soul-self from your mind-self. In general, the results of meditative practices help with focus and clarity, reduced anxiety and the ability to make life decisions free from the knee jerk reactions of our emotional states.

The definition of meditation and the techniques used are vast and numerous. The oldest historical traditions include Hinduism with contemplation and yoga, for the pure awareness of self as separate from the mind (the self within one's self). Buddhism uses breathwork, contemplation and visualization for awakening and the achievement of nirvana. Jainism's aim of meditation is salvation and freedom of the soul. Japanese Zazen uses a form of seated meditation for insight into the nature of existence. Taoism uses contemplative concentration, mindfulness and visualization, for insight and Qi cultivation. These are embedded in practices like Qigong, martial arts, Daoyin and Taijiquan (shadow boxing).

There does not seem to be any modern agreement

on what constitutes mediation. The ancient practices have spread and evolved greatly around the world as each teacher and student impressed their own styles on inherited practices. Meditation however has not always been just part of the eastern philosophies and religions. It has always been a central tool in pagan ceremonies and indigenous traditional practices. It has also been an a intricate part of all the world's monotheistic religions in the form of Christian prayers like the "Our Father" or Catholic "Rosary", Islamic Sufi "Dhikr" or Muslim "Salah or Salat" and the Jewish "Hitbodedut". Mediation here as being the vehicle used on a path to an encounter with God.

The word "meditation" comes from the Latin verb "medatari" which means "to think, contemplate, devise and ponder". It does not need to be scripted by the rules of a particular eastern practice or a modern day religion. However, the ancient practices do have an edge on how to achieve the desired results. It is said that the mediation practice itself should not be the goal. While the habit of meditating is relaxing and calming, those serious about meditation say the desired outcome should be enlightenment, self knowledge, wisdom, peace and a connection with the divine universal force.

A note of warning however. Mediation is not for everyone. Those who are suffering trauma (this is a growing number of people) meditation may concentrate the pain. When still in the throes of the flight or fight response, long after an incident, sitting still in reflection will not be possible. Even trying may exacerbate the feelings of failure. Be kind to yourself, know you are loved by the Creator, even if it is difficult to find any form of love or kindness in human form. This will pass.

During the interim healing journey, just examine any swings in emotion for the thoughts that triggered the eruption. Then try to reprogram those negative or self-debasing narratives, with loving and good thoughts about yourself. Re-wiring, undoing and retraining the mind and healing the heart, takes time. Mediation is for those who are fishing for deep and hidden shadows and want to expand their soul-peace. For those who are suffering trauma, no digging is needed. That darkness is in your face. Instead try breathwork and affirmations.

Vocal Toning

Using your voice and chanting is an effective way to boost your mind's energy. In Qigong there are sounds for every organ system. You can, however, just make whatever sounds you want and feel the humming vibration move to different areas of the body. One good routine is to visualize an energy ball over three major energy centres of the body. The upper one is between the base of the skull and the third eye. The middle one is in the centre of the chest (Heart). The lower one is in the interior of the body, below the navel towards the lower back area.

At the same time of the visualization at each centre, vocalize sounds for each area ("Weng" for head, "Ar" for heart area and "Hong" for the lower abdomen). Place your hands with fingers touching and palms facing toward the body in front of each energy centre at the same time as the chanting and visualization. It is important for the palms to face the body, not away from the body to direct the energy from your heart to your hands and then inward. Being grateful activates the heart, so finish each centre by repeating thank you to your body, yourself and your higher power.

Breathwork

Breathwork or Pranayama, is thousands of years old and originates from India and China. It is a practice of consciously breathing with awareness and intent. The techniques focus on deep breathing in a way that triggers the parasympathetic nervous system to turn off the flight/fright sympathetic responses. The result is a sense of relaxation, reduced blood pressure, increased energy, a sense of calmness and a feeling of being centred or grounded. The increased energy is the result of higher oxygenation of the body, better sleep, immunity and better overall functioning of all our body systems.

When a person is stressed, the breaths they take are shallow and more rapid. The human flight or fight response triggers the altered breathing to increase the intake of oxygen, in a fearful situation. However shallow breathing over time actually restricts the amount of oxygen that the body can absorb. Many people breathe like this, most of the time and it becomes a feedback loop telling the body, it is stressed. So the anxiety that causes the shallow breathing then triggers the body into thinking there is a threat, even after that has long passed. The results include panic attacks, asthma, irregular heartbeat, ringing in the ears, dizziness and tingling in the extremities.

Paying attention to and controlling the breath is now an accepted tool within the field of health and wellness. There are now many various techniques for deep breathing and increasing the oxygen supply to the body. The results are different depending on the technique used and can range from relaxation to an altered state of consciousness.

Breathwork can also be used to help people to move past emotional and mental blockages to alleviate the causes of anger or depression, for example. It does that by changing the frequencies of our energetic brain waves that range between 35+Hz (gamma) used for high focus to 0.5-4.0Hz (delta) when in a deep relaxed state or sleep. Beta waves of 12-35Hz are where most of us function in our daily life. Alpha waves at 8-12Hz occur when we are in a relaxed state. However theta waves of 4-8Hz are where we are deeply relaxed, intuitive and creative. The delta waves are most common in children and young adults and are the slowest waves associated with regenerative sleep and healing.

Learning to breathe slowly with intention takes practice and can feel very awkward at first. A common technique is the 4-7-8 (inhale on 4 counts, hold for 7 counts, exhale on 8 counts). The slow deep breaths should allow the belly to expand and is also called "belly breathing". Breathing is also a form of meditation and goes in hand with that practice. It can help you connect your physical body with your inner-self, mind-thoughts and your spirit-self. Some say that the slower you breathe, the longer you live.

For breath is life and if you breathe well you will live long on earth. - Sanskrit proverb

Mental Frequencies

If everything around us emits invisible waves that affect our energy, how can we protect ourselves? The people we surround ourselves with and the environment we find ourselves in, can either deplete or energize us. Our mind can also trigger emotions that can cause us to feel upset or stressed. Therefore fostering good thoughts, seeking peace of mind and taking charge of the brain-mind, is key.

The brain is a powerful, complex organ that allows us to think, plan, remember, analyze and strategize. It is a centralized message centre for chemical and electrical stimuli both transmitting and receiving. A strong, clear working mind can solve problems, innovate and set us apart as a superior organism. The mind can also cause problems. It can lead us astray if we believe everything it tells us. Ideas swimming around in our subconscious self, have a large impact on how we behave and how we feel about ourselves. Anyone who has attempted meditation, becomes acutely aware of the avalanche of out-of-control thoughts, lurking in the subconscious.

Our mind is not who we are and we need to be aware that our mind is a tool we need to command.

The mind can actually lead us astray if we are not careful. Taking charge of what goes on in the brain requires introspection. The mind does not know everything. Careful analysis allows us to check in and pull back the curtains of what is going on in the mind. It is also helpful to cultivate balanced thinking, by fostering attention to other body signals like emotions, body language, gut feel and intuition.

Thoughts create feelings. Identifying emotions that are disproportionate to a situation, becomes a clue to an imbalance. Sometimes you will find a rogue idea has been unintentionally planted in our mind by an outside force. Like a long gone teacher saying, "you will never amount to anything", for example. Sometimes people intentionally say hurtful things to harm our mental well-being. Especially when vulnerable, we must guard ourselves against people who consistently mess with our minds. We also have to make sure we do not internalize the words and allow the trauma to negatively affect us. Having strong and healthy boundaries is important to protect our well-being.

Meditation, journaling and talk therapy with someone we trust, can help us keep a check on our mental health. We can also monitor what we watch on television, read on the internet, what books we read and what movies we watch. We all know someone who loves to read crime stories and watch the news, especially CNN. Then they don't know why they feel depressed and anxious. All that gore, especially this pandemic news, has a profound effect on all of us.

It is good to be aware of how the information,

inputs and people around you are affecting you. Balance the need to know, with how you are feeling about the content of what you are watching or reading. For example if while watching the news, you feel stress butterflies in the stomach or a growing sense of anger or depression, stop and switch to something cheerful. Ranting at the TV or inappropriately responding to others on social media is a good sign that a change of focus is needed. Keeping some level of awareness about how you are feeling and watching the signals of your body, when you are engaged in activities, or around people, goes a long way in protecting mental health.

Instead of just protecting one's self from harmful mind-energy, it is a good practice to seek out people who are like minded, who understand and respect us. Laughing and spending time with those who uplift us, is an especially important way to gather healing frequencies. Our own positive self-talk, and putting ourselves in places with people who give us good feedback, raises and smooths-out our mind frequencies into sinusoidal waves with healthy energy.

Affirmations

While mediation helps with the voluntary control of thought, affirmations are a way of reprogramming the involuntary wanderings of the mind. They are also a powerful tool for aligning with universal frequencies. Whether we like it or not, or if we are even aware of it, our thoughts tend to have a life of their own. These wayward thoughts have been fed to us since birth and have been etched into our memories like a well wired circuit board.

One way to combat negative limiting thoughts are to repeat the opposite uplifting beliefs. Then say these things over and over, ruminating on the positive words, until the new thoughts are understood and make more sense. The repetition of the positive ideas and the internal arguments for and against them, creates a whole dissertation in favour of the positive mindset. Eventually these better thoughts overthrow the unhealthy wiring because we believe the new thoughts and are inspired to live up to them.

Affirmations can be created to have on hand when needed. Remind yourself of your successes in overcoming scary situations in the past. Make a list of past acts of courage and bravery demonstrating how you can face anything that comes your way. Think back over your life at your accomplishments. Take an inventory of your good qualities. Look at all the times when you were able to overcome hard times and difficult challenges. Have these lists ready and be ready to recite them over and over each time you discover an unhealthy thought pattern. By doing this, you are pre-armed to address the negative thought until it becomes powerless and fades away.

I am loved, I am respected,
I am healthy, I am healed;
I am validated, I am vindicated,
I am exonerated, I am free;
I am one with the universe,
and the universe is in me. - SG Williams

Affirmations can also be put on vision boards, as pictures of what we want to achieve. Thinking about goals and desires and then committing them to a visual representation, helps clarify what we want. The exercise of creating the board is a way to focus on our desired vision of the future. Then as we view the vision board, day after day, the visual repetition not only affirms what we want, but helps us align and resonate with particular outcomes that make them happen. This synchronicity with the universe makes us co-creators of our world. Each picture on the board will flow into our reality one by one, just as we had dreamed they would.

6 Spirit - Soul

The foundation of a healthy spiritual life cannot be described easily. It is enough to say that if you are curious and are seeking to understand your sub-conscience life and looking for the authentic you, that is a good foundational baseline. Our spiritual beliefs are based on our education, culture, assumptions and experiences. Finding within yourself, threads of kindness, love and goodness and fostering those virtues combined with good intentions, is all you need for empowered healing. Healing is about the process of becoming whole, balanced and being your true self in the world. Seeking to heal and be healed will help you find your way.

Tips on Spiritual Clutter

...Spiritual Clutter:...(it) obscures our vision... hinders us on our path. Each of us has a life purpose...Clearing clutter in all forms allows our

original purpose…to re-surface…to clear the debris that prevents us from connecting with our Higher Self. - Karen Kingston

Not only is it important to keep your house tidy so good energy can circulate, we need to keep our bodies, our mind, our thoughts, our relationships, our consciences and our intentions tidy. Here are Karen's suggestions:

- Adopt healthy eating habits that can give you that perfect bowel movement to help with physical clutter in our bodies.

- Write to-do lists and tie up the loose ends of tasks, to provide up-time for focus on the important things. It help clear up mental clutter.

- Examine your eccentricities. For example why everything in your home has ducks or cats on it, or why you can't throw out something you don't need or use? The investigation could help identify blockages, or unmet needs, to clear emotional clutter.

- Accept others for who they are and refrain from judging, criticizing, worrying, gossiping and the mental chatter that makes us unhappy. This clears psychological clutter.

- Seek relationships that uplift us. Forgive others to help recover the lost bits of our spirit. This makes us more complete and clears spiritual clutter.

- Expect good things, be grateful and trust we

will be cared for. This will manifest it into reality. This clears clutter from our connection to the universe and our higher power.

When we throw out the physical clutter, we clear our minds. When we throw out the mental clutter, we clear our souls. - Gail Blanke

Letting Go

When we can't find that peaceful mind-space, introspection and attempting meditation, is very good at making us aware of the mind-chatter and emotional trauma that we try to avoid, or just don't realize is there. When we do an examination of what is being dredged up from the bottom of our mental and emotional pools, it is important to not only identify the clutter, but to dispose of it somehow. This is easier said than done. But if we want to be healthy, this is truly important.

There is always a root cause to what is causing us spiritual discomfort. Guilt, shame and anger often stay long after events have passed. Wiping the memories away or avoiding them with busyness, does not remove the emotional scars. To resolve this and work towards letting go, let the emotions wash over you as they arise. Do this in a safe place. Don't bury them but give them a small amount of time and recognition. Lean into the uncomfortable feeling and try to understand them. Then let the emotions dissipate or give yourself a time limit for the rumination. Over time their negative power will decline.

Psychologists generally define forgiveness as a conscious, deliberate decision to release feelings of resentment or vengeance toward a person or group who has harmed you, regardless of whether they actually deserve your forgiveness. ...Forgiveness does not mean forgetting, nor does it mean condoning or excusing offences..

Forgiveness is a powerful state of being that can facilitate a peaceful spirit. Forgiveness allows us to let go of the hurts, remorse and anger. This action ultimately allows us to forget, move on and connect to our soul-self. However it is not easy to do unless you understand that forgiveness is not something you do for the perpetrator. It is a gift to yourself. What they did may always remain unconscionable in your mind. You may want to punish them by holding on to the hurt but it really only damages your own spirit. They will ultimately be accountable somehow, some way to what they have done. At the very least, what they did has damaged them too, even if they never acknowledge it.

Instead of getting revenge by reciprocating, the best revenge you can muster is to forgive, let go and live life well. Don't allow them to live rent free in your mind. I heard an interview with the Dalai Lama when he was asked how he survived the dangers of the invasion of Nepal by the Chinese. He responded that the physical danger was not as great as the spiritual one. His greatest danger was/is in avoiding hating the Chinese for what they did. In the same way the damage of past hurts can be mitigated when we forgive, the real harm to us is spiritually, when we don't.

Forgiveness does not mean that you condone what was done, or admit to them and others that it was OK. It does not mean that you forget what happened or that you don't continue to have negative feelings and be upset by what they did. It means that you don't let the event and the other person control you to the point of being consumed by it. Forgiveness means that you progressively manage it in a way that it does not affect your peace of mind. You need to place the event into a particular envelope, seal it and place it in one of the minor folders, in the filing cabinet of memories that live in your mind.

It is most important in the process of acceptance and letting go, is that we forgive ourselves. Be kind to yourself, admit how you feel and then remind yourself of your overall goodness and all the things you did get right. Accept them as part of who you are and remember the growth that always comes through mistakes.

Scientists at the University of St. Andrews highlighted the importance of being able to let go in their research about forgiveness. They showed that those participants who were willing to forgive their transgressor were more likely to be able to forget what happened. For this very reason, it's so important to be able to let go and forgive that we can move on with our life.

Check the Ego

When we spend a lot of time overthinking, we can lose perspective and control over our mind's imagination. Our mental creations can give the ego free reign. The mind creates a false sense of who we are as unique, special, important and separate from others and nature. It ignores the idea that we are all connected. It takes input from the world around it, to feed that separateness and sense of importance. Anything that threatens self importance, is the enemy and it breeds conflict with what we truly feel. The ego is an artificial construct of the mind and its need to dominate, makes us unhappy and casts a shadow over our authentic self.

The ego can also be overly sober about everything. A person who takes themselves too seriously, is not able to enjoy life and have fun (maybe perhaps at the expense of others). This can depress a desirable elevated vibrational state, not just in themselves, but in everyone around them. Such an ego cannot laugh at itself. That is not healthy when we know that laughter is good for us. It is a great way to raise the frequency of our vibrations. However, laughing at or in the presence of someone who has a big ego, is not safe. Just the slightest incongruence with their belief in respect due and hierarchical position, will be aggressively challenged.

There is no limit to what an over inflated ego will do, to defend its own sense of self, no matter how false it is. The ego is the great pretender and the one it fools is the person it rules. It is a good idea to find a way to protect yourself from your own ego. Try to stay off the proverbial pedestal by not climbing up it in the first place, you will get knocked off by somebody, somehow, eventually. Socializing with friends and family is a great way to keep the ego in check. People you love and trust will let you know if you become unbalanced and provide the needed reality check. However, nobody is ego free. It is part of the human condition.

In the spiritual sense, an unrestrained ego denies the existence of the true self. This robs us of our power, by disconnecting us from the universal source. The lack of synchronicity with our divine nature, creates havoc in the world around us. We do not resonate with it. We feel alone and alien in the world as a result. En masse, this leads to every evil we see in the world today, from injustice to our environmental crisis. The ego and its ramifications are one aspect of the universal divine force. We need to cultivate our true selves, to restore balance to ourselves, others and the world.

Tap into Spirit

Energy is the message sent by vibrational frequencies that communicate with us in profound ways. We have a spirit energy that can detect issues and is sending us messages. It allows us to sense things that we can't understand with our minds. It can tell our cells to heal themselves or cause us to impact and be affected by the energy around us. That event you just have a gut feel about and really don't want to go to, just don't go. Over time you will start to see the wisdom of your spirit.

Our heart spirit also tells us what we need to do, where we need to go, or who we need to be with. It is sometimes harder to understand. It is like the heart has another mind. I know that the gut has been labelled as the second brain. However many believe that the heart is the seat of the soul. The heart-mind connection has been proven to activate a powerful radiance of compassionate energy. However the heart houses the Shen, controls the Shen and is the emperor or ruler. Even though spirits are housed in all the organs, the Five-Shen together, makes up our soul. Therefore the heart is the supreme brain.

Chinese Medicine considers Shen to be one of the three treasures that constitute life: Jing, the essence; Qi, the life force; and Shen, the spirit. TCM views the spirit as an integral part of our health and our well-being and cultivation of the spirit is considered essential for health maintenance.

...

Chinese masters say it is through Shen that we radiate ourselves into the world. This spiritual radiance manifests as our wisdom, emotional well-being, and ability to see all sides of an issue. Shen refers to that aspect of our being that looks to the universe around us, and is not focused on emotions. Shen draws our attention to the divine. It contributes to wisdom, virtue, and calmness, and maintains our whole being in order. - Diane Joswick

The heart is also the biggest energy centre of the body that grows when we think about the needs of others, or are connected to your higher power, God or the universe. That heart energy radiates from the hands and allows you to heal yourself and others, using visualizations and detailed directed intention. When supported by like minded others, such intention is powerful.

But how do you connect to that spirit within you? Where does it live? Could that same energy oscillating at a particular frequency of form, that we cannot see, that permeates our being and communicates with us, be part of the same thing we call God, goddess, higher power, Tao or Brahman? Perhaps it is only when we resonate and synchronize with these frequencies, that we even know they exist? Maybe the macrocosm that is the universe, is the same extension of the microcosm that exists within our bodies, cells, molecules and atoms, just on different scales?

What are the portals, the ways or doors we use to find our union with the divine? Spiritual practices of all forms are there to help us resonate at the frequencies that allow us to synchronize and communicate, with the omnipotent power that is already part of us. Meditation, prayer, fasting, yoga, penance, mind altering herbs, physical extremes such as walking pilgrimages or sweat lodges are a few examples. Spiritual teachers, Gurus, Shamans and Saints are there to help us make sense of all these practices and guide us towards and through the portals.

Another gateway to the spirit is through gratitude. This uses the mind to open the heart portal. Some say this is the highest of all virtues. Others say it is thankfulness with a sense of wonder. Gratitude is something you can take action and control by the way you look at your life and the events in it. You can tune yourself into being grateful with your mind. Then once that gateway is opened, our heart opens, then love and compassion naturally flow from that. Compassion is powerful. It does not stop at just allowing us to understand and feel what others are going through, it moves us to make things better.

Tapping into Spirit is ultimately merging ourselves with the universal power of creation in order to resonate with all that is. Eastern mystics believe that we are all an expression of the one higher power. Jesus himself indicated this when he said that as the children of God, we would do even greater things than He. Christian saints and mystics discovered a union with the divine in their individual spiritual experiences. Indigenous people have always seen themselves as spirit beings, dressed as humans. In all these aspects of belief, the divine is who we are and we continue in some form after death.

It makes sense that we are as much a part of the natural world as the creatures and plants around us. That if they thrive without all the complications of a modern society, so can we. All religions and philosophies have common threads, in that they all say we are spirit beings connected to a universal power and that there is life after death. A world like ours, that is so beautiful, ordered, mindbogglingly complex, with purposes for every organism in the grand web of life, could not just happen by chance.

If we possess the spirit of the universe in every cell, that is also connected to the universe that surrounds us, this is a connection we need to explore. This totality of being whole and being well, is the solid foundation we need to build on, to better heal ourselves and others. The more we resonate with our true nature, others and the natural world around us, the more balanced we become. Being aware of our emotions helps us to keep our mind and heart in touch with spirit. Keeping our ego in check, forgiveness, releasing strong emotions, finding things to be grateful for, accepting difficulties as life-lessons and seeing others as your-other-self, builds compassion and connection to your heart. The connection to the heart is a connection to our spirit soul.

"You are not IN the universe, you ARE the universe, an intrinsic part of it. Ultimately, you are not a person, but the focal point where the universe is becoming conscious of itself. What an amazing miracle." - Eckhart Tolle

7 Healing Methods

Healing and developing a spiritual life takes place over the entire duration of one's life. Sometimes it is one step forward and two steps back, followed by a giant leap head again. Life provides us with many challenges. However anyone can actively facilitate healing for themselves, others and the world, no matter where you are in your journey. There are some techniques I learned from my own healing practice and years of research that I found to be powerful. I used these in my one on one practice with clients and then started teaching these in groups. Healing in groups is powerful and effective, if there is mutual understanding and respect.

These methods take much of the information presented in this book and concentrate them into one active healing session. The methods presented here do not have to be done in exactly the same way as I have presented them. Living a good life, the best one can, raising the energy in the body, mind and spirit with detailed, focused intention, provides the greatest healing energy. Add to this a mind-heart connection filled with a compassionate presence, completes the key elements to empowered healing.

Prepare

Have everyone in the circle, focus on the immediate space as it is cleared with good frequencies. The intention here is to clear and purify the space of negative energy and emotions. You can also use the various techniques below in any way that makes sense to you.

SOUND: As people gather for the healing circle, employing healing sounds. Music toned to nature is a good way to elevate the vibration of the room. Singing, chanting and toning sounds have a direct impact not just on the space but the person creating the vibrations. You can also have one person play singing bowls, tuning forks, or have a drum circle where everyone can participate with a percussion instrument of their choice. Use drums and drumming, tuning forks, singing bowls, gongs, healing music and/or chanting for as long as you like.

COLOURS: Depending on who is in the room and what their needs are, you might want to highlight particular colours. The root chakra at the base of the torso vibrates with red and represents our sense of stability and security in the world. The sacral, above the root and below the naval, vibrates orange and is our creative and sexual energy. Above that the solar plexus is yellow, governing our willpower and self esteem. The heart centre is green and is all about relationships. The throat chakra is light blue and represents our ability to communicate. The third-eye between the eyebrows, is indigo blue and our intuition. The crown chakra, just above the top of the head, is purple, our higher self and our connection to the divine.

If someone was having an issue with or wanted to strengthen any of these areas, wearing the corresponding colour or seeing it through a tinted lens, can help improve that weakness. The key is to expose the group to the frequencies of that energy centre that might need extra attention. Also to keep in mind some studies show that hue, tint and brightness of colours triggers emotion and has a physiological effect on how we feel. Brighter more saturated colours evoke positive emotions than muted hues.

PURE ESSENTIAL OILS (Aromatherapy): Pure essential oils are more expensive than fragrances, but you only need a few drops at a time. Make sure the oils are in a dark bottle that carries the Latin name, the common name, the supplier name, the country of origin, the organic stamp and any other additive or oils, if diluted. Unlike chemical synthetic scents, essential oils do not have negative side effects. They are very balanced. However safety is important. Do not overuse one oil. Putting a few drops of oil in a diffuser or in a burner with water to evaporate it, goes a long way. For a healing circle fir and black spruce are good scents for grounding. Then adding frankincense is a nice mixture, because it will enhance a meditative state. To enhance positive thoughts and emotions you could use cardamom and orange.

CRYSTALS: Amethyst is exceptionally high in vibration and is good at clearing rooms of any negative energies. Its purple colour corresponds to the crown chakra that connects us to our intuition. It is particularly good to have for healing rituals. Citrine can be used to strengthen positive energy. Quartz is good for amplifying the vibrations of all other crystals and for enhancing a connection to the higher self.

Open Circle

This preparation creates a sacred circle that is delineated in a way that honours your own experiences and beliefs. The purpose of this is to foster a safe place of good and clear intention, without interference or distraction.

Have everyone close their eyes and visualize a flow of energy moving in the direction of the earth's rotation from west to east. After a minute or so, speak aloud that "only love may enter this circle". Clear your thoughts and become present in the now. Allow all negativity to drift away. Then ask aloud, for a blessing from the source of all life and for the support of spirit allies (use your own belief system here). This may involve a call for the blessing of the unseen helpers, the setting of directions of the elements and an invitation to the eternal source of life or ancestors, power animals, spirits, angels or saints, depending on your culture. This circle remains until after the end of the healing session, when it is formally dissolved by the expression of thanks to all attendees seen and unseen.

A - BODY

1. Increase Qi

Starting with Qigong. This is a physically active, therapeutic movement that combines mediation, breathwork, visualizations and sounds. It is a way to gather and harness energy from nature while preserving your life force, ensuring the energy is balanced and flows smoothly through the body. I like to use the Eight Brocade which is a well known, ancient set of movements. There are many examples of online videos showing slightly different versions. Repeat these movements:

1. Warm up the lower Dantien: Between your kidneys, below your navel, by swinging your arms clockwise then counterclockwise while hitting your lower back and then lower front abdomen.

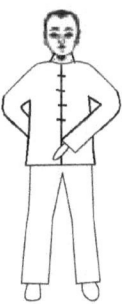

2. Holding Hands to Heaven: Gather Qi from the lower front of the body, as if scooping it up from the ground and placing it into your abdomen. Then with outstretched arms, reach up to heaven with palms

facing upward. Then turn the palms downward and draw hands down as if pulling Qi into the head.

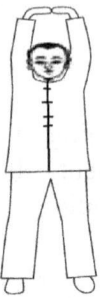

3. Separating Heaven and Earth: Draw hands up from the earth, palms up, as if picking up a ball of Qi. Then push one hand above (palm up) and one below (palm down) as if separating the Qi ball. Then alternate the arms and repeat.

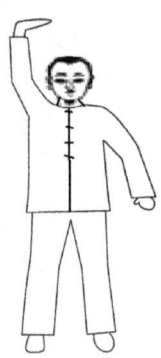

4. Drawing the Bow: With legs in an open stance, knees bent in a deep lunge. Face one side, pull hands together, to the chest and then separate them. One arm points to the side as if aiming the arrow. The other arm reaches out and pulls back the string. Then swing to the other side to do it again.

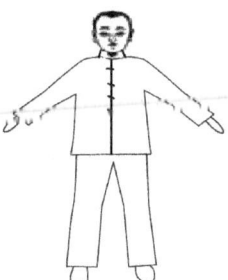

5. Wise Owl Looks Back: Standing with knees bent and arms to the side, turn side to side moving the head backwards as far as possible.

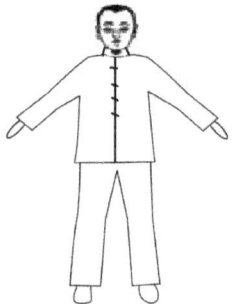

6. Sway the Head and Wag the Tail: With legs open, bend at the waist towards the earth and swing in an arc from one side to another. Move upward to one side, back down to the centre and up to the other side.

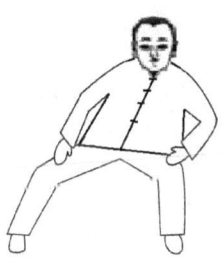

7. Holding Back and Ankles: Bending forward, trace the arms from the lower back down the back of the legs to the ankles. Hold them, then bring them up the front of the legs, up the body and reach to the sky. Then draw Qi down from the sky to the body and repeat.

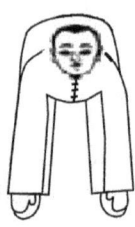

8. Punching: Legs apart, bent in a wide lunge position, palms clenched facing the upper chest. Then quickly punch outward with one arm and turn fist down. As that arm pulls back into the chest, punch outward with the other arm.

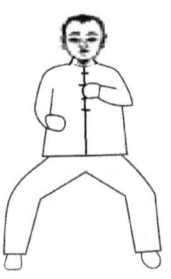

9. Shake Up: Lean forward then slowly stand tall and then on to tip toes. Then plunk yourself down on your heels. Bend backwards then slowly straighten up and then up on the toes. Then plunk yourself down to shake your body again.

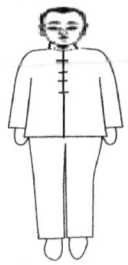

2. Activate Meridians

Instead of using needles to stimulate acupuncture points, we can use pressure (acupressure) and tapping. The points furthest away from the organs are often the most powerful. This means there are many accessible points along the hands, feet, arms and legs. The pressure and tapping should be fairly firm. The points are named after the meridian on which they are located, followed by a number.

Below are locations of 6 sets of points on the 12 primary meridians. They were chosen so that the thumb and middle finger can put pressure on two points at the same time. By pressing these points in the order listed, you can open the meridians in the way Qi naturally flows through the body.

1. Start with Lung 10 (Lu10, Yugi or Fish Border) and Large Intestine 4 (Li4, Hegu or Junction Valley) by grabbing the inside and outside of the hand below the thumb.

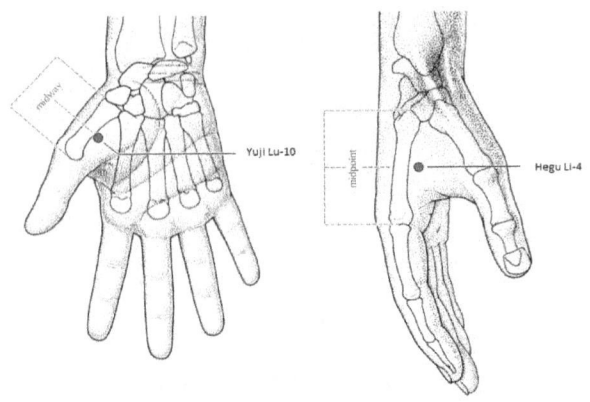

2. Follow with Stomach 36 (St36, Zusanli or Leg Three Miles) and Spleen 9 (Sp9, Yinlingquan or Yin Mound Spring) by grabbing the inside and outside of the leg below the knee.

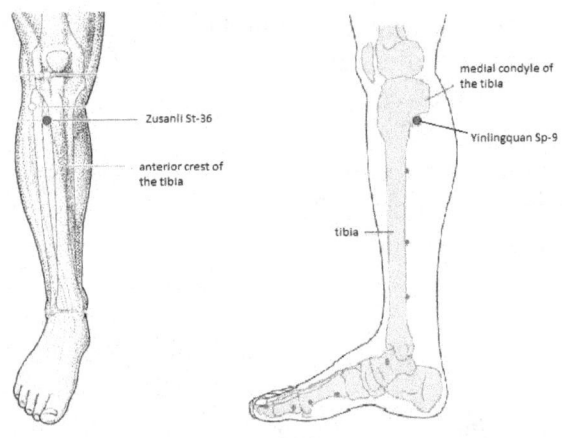

3. Then Heart 7 (Ht7, Shenmen or Spirit Gate) and Small Intestine 6 (Si6, Yanglao or Support The Aged) by grabbing the underside and topside of the outer wrist.

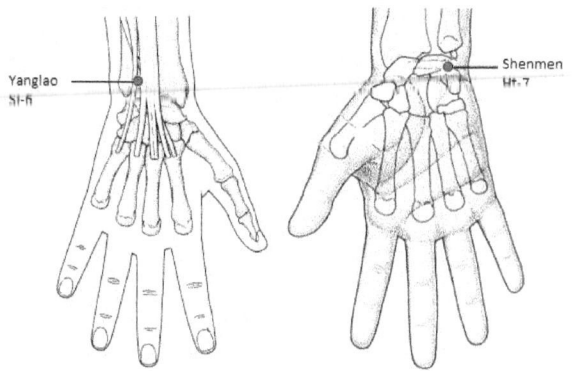

4. The fourth set of points are Bladder 60 (Bl60, Kunlun or Kunlun Mountains) and Kidney 3 (Ki3, Taixi or Great Stream) by grabbing either side of the ankle above the heel and below the ankle bone.

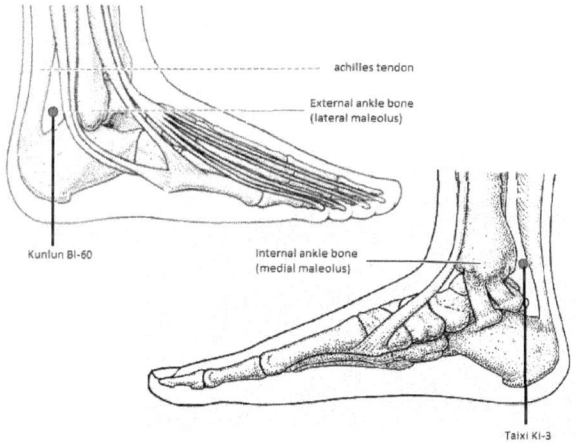

5. The fifth set is Pericardium 6 (Pc6, Neiguan or Inner Pass) and Triple Warmer or San Jiao 5 (Tw or Sj5, Waiguan or Outer Pass), inside and outside of the lower arm two thumb widths above the wrist.

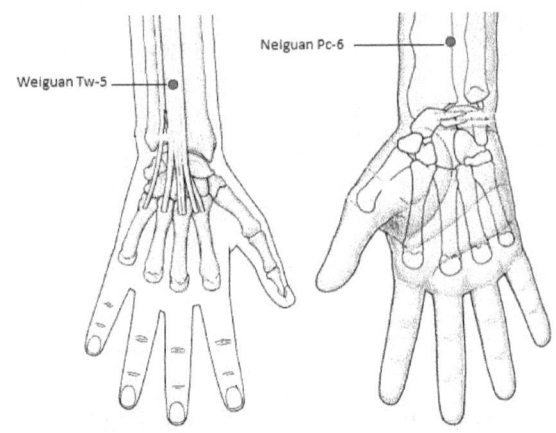

6. Finally, 6th are Gallbladder 40 (Gb40, Qiuxu or Mound of Ruins) and Liver 4 (Lv4, Zhongfeng or Middle Margin) by pinching the two points on top of the foot between the ankle bones.

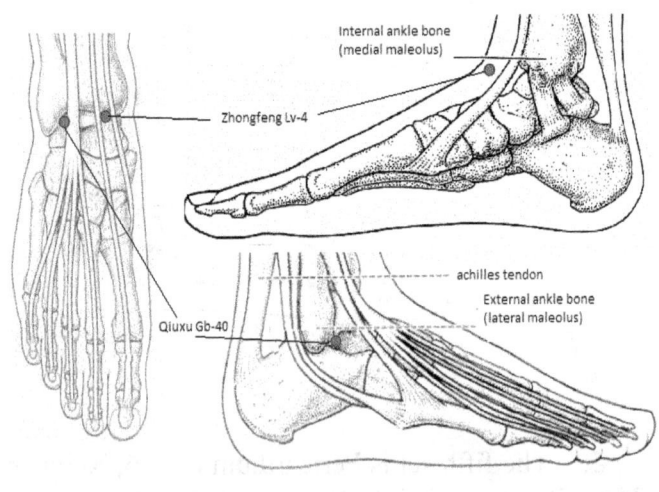

After the acupressure, use EFT to calm the emotions and improve mind-clarity, use the Emotional Freedom Technique by tapping on each of the 9 points.

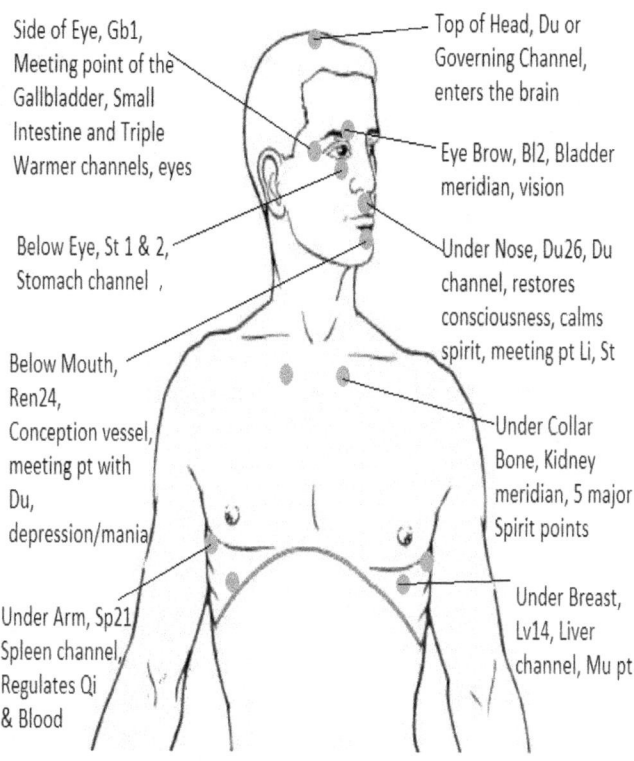

3. Direct Qi

There are 3 main energy centres of the body. The Lower Dantien (between kidneys and 3 fingers below the naval), the Middle Dantian at the heart (centre of chest and the torso) and the Upper Dantian, the Third

Eye (centre of the forehead and at the base of the back of the skull or pineal gland area). The hands are also a strong centre of energy emission and can be used with visualization and intention, to direct the Qi.

The hands can be used to both concentrate the Qi and in cases of too much, can also be used to dissipate excess energy. By holding one hand near the area of excess, palm inward and the second hand away from the body, palm outward, the Qi is directed away from the body. Here, we want to place both hands over the 3 energy centres with palms facing inward to increase the Qi in these energy centres.

Along with the visualizations and hand positions below, it is important to connect the heart and mind. We do this by being grateful and thankful. This seals the completion of Qi manifestation.

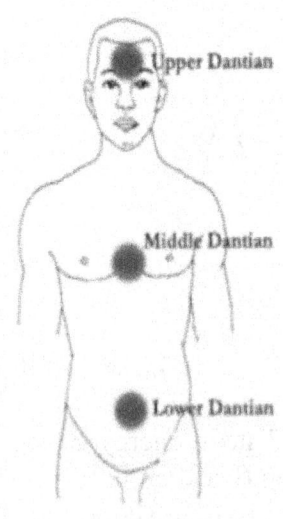

For each energy centre, starting with the lower one and moving up to the crown:

1. Hold hands over the area, palms inward, breathe calmly.

2. Visualize a golden ball of light entering the energy centre.

3. Ask for healing in these areas from your higher power and spiritual team of allies.

4. Visualize the area as strong, vital, healthy and healed.

5. Out loud or silently, tell your team that you Love them.

6. Out loud or silently, with gratitude, Thank 3 beings (your body, your spirit allies, your higher power) for your healing.

MIND

4. Calm Mind

As you have increased the flow, concentrated the Qi and directed the energy, now is the time to harness the mind. You want to be able to give the energy clear and direct instructions which take clarity and focus. Next you want to balance the 3 main energy centres. In the Indian Vedas, there are 7 major energy centres. I have lumped these into the 3 we are using here based in TCM. The goal here is to achieve a calm mind.

For each energy centre, we will use toning with vocalized sounds, and breathwork to balance the vibration. We can also combine colours and sounds from other instruments. Singing bowls, with frequencies that correlate to the chakras, can be played and the corresponding colours can be placed over the energy centres, as added options.

1. Starting with the Lower Dantien, chanting the sound of the word "Hong" will create vibrations in this region. The colours of the lower area are red (root chakra) and orange (sacral chakra).

2. For the Middle Dantian, the word "Ar" activates the central Heart energy centre. The colours that correspond to this are yellow (solar plexus chakra) and green (heart chakra).

3. For the Upper Dantian, the word is "Weng". This corresponds to the Throat, Third Eye and Crown chakras with colours light blue, dark blue and purple respectively.

As you chant the words, feel the vibrations resonate in these energy centres. Feel these areas open and change. This should begin to calm and open the mind as you transition from toning sounds into breathwork.

At this point change focus to the breath. A common technique is the 4-7-8 (inhale on 4 counts, hold for 7 counts, exhale on 8 counts). Some like to call it "belly breathing" because of the slow deep breaths that let the belly expand. Others like to count to 6 as the lungs expand to the very bottom of the stomach (belly), hold it and then just let go so that the breath just falls out, creating a rush of exhaled air that is not forced, but natural.

Here for The Code, slow down to deep breaths by counting to 6 as the lungs expand to the very bottom of the belly. Hold it for 3 counts, then let go and let the breath just fall out as follows:

1. Inhale to fill the belly. Exhale.

2. Inhale to fill the belly. Exhale.

3. Inhale to fill the heart. Exhale.

4. Inhale to let the breath stir the emotions. Exhale the insecure thoughts and old traumas.

5. Inhale to melt into your consciousness. Exhale as you meld with the universe.

6. Inhale to fill your heart with gratitude. Exhale your thanks to all that support you.

5. Clear Thoughts

While in stillness and after the breathing activity, we then flow naturally into several moments of personal mediation. Sitting comfortably, focus on a particular object, sound or your breath. As you encounter mind-chatter, the task is to become centred enough to put aside the thoughts and not be controlled by them. As each thought comes into view and the sphere of awareness, acknowledge it and then let it pass. Take care not to dwell on it. Put it aside for later if you can. Whatever emotion may arise, just let it wash over you. The goal is to achieve a mentally clear state where we can be mindful and aware.

Sit quietly in your own personal form of meditation. Remain still and quiet until everyone in the room has finished.

6. Direct Mind

We become what we think about, and as Emerson reminded us: "The ancestor to every action is a thought." As these thoughts of plenitude and excessive sufficiency become your way of thinking, the all-creating force to which you're always connected will begin to work with you, in harmony with your thoughts... - Wayne Dyer

Once the mind is clearer, we want to direct our minds to positive thoughts. We will create and repeat positive statements about ourselves to challenge and overcome any lingering, self-sabotaging, chatter. What those statements are, depends on the person but I will provide an example below. The affirmations should be repeated aloud or to yourself a minimum of 3 times. Repeating them helps you believe them. This causes them to manifest.

I am safe,

I am happy,
I am healthy.
The universe loves me,
I have everything I need,
to heal myself, others and the world.

SPIRIT

7. Set Intention

If you are in a group, each person should have a healing intention for themselves or another person. You can also pick a person to pair up with and share your needs with each other. The group may also be there for the healing needs of one person who has shared their needs with the group.

Gather an understanding of the healing need, using as much of the details as the person is willing to share, including anatomy and physiology, if possible. Because of privacy, you can still formulate effective intentions with less detail. From what you have, formulate a specific tailored intention for yourself or another person. That intention should address the details of the problem and what the end goal will look like. Envision the end healthy state, describe it and feel it. Depending on the situation, the statement of intention can be said out loud or silently and privately.

8. Open Heart

The next step is to connect the mind's intentions to an open heart by tapping into spirit. Here we use a specific scripted heart mediation* to open the heart to compassion and love. Have everyone close their eyes as this meditation is read out loud:

Heart Meditation:

Breathe in and breathe out and just let go of any old stuff. Put one hand on your heart and one hand on your belly. And as you breathe quietly, notice how comforting that feels. And as you release yesterday and even this moment, you allow your full attention to come into this day, this hour, this time. Turn your full attention to this wonderful, wonderful day,

Imagine yourself in the centre of a circle made up of the most loving beings you've met. Receive the love of those who love you. Experience yourself as the recipient of the energy, attention, care, and regard of all of these beings in your circle of love. Open yourself up to receiving love. There's nothing special that you need to do to deserve this kind of acknowledgement or care. It's simply because you exist.

Send loving care to the people in your circle. You can allow that quality of loving kindness and compassion and care you feel coming toward you to flow right back out to the circle and then toward all beings everywhere, so that what you receive, you transform into giving. Let your heart open and make room for all the good of the Universe to come in.

With a hand on heart connect to your inner self, higher self. Then connect with the inner-selves of those around you and while holding that connection consider the attributes of the other person that you appreciate and are grateful for.

You may feel an overpowering love pour out for this person, that goes beyond the capacity of human love. When you see them as the unique beautiful shining star that they are, you know you have tapped into the energy of the creator. You are no longer alone, the spirit team is in your midst helping. You are one and in a state of resonance with all there is.

Then with an open heart, repeat the detailed intention. As you do, see it manifest as if it has already happened. Watch the pain disappear, function return, vitality glow and feel the joy of freedom from the ailment. Watch the person dance around in perfect health.

When you're connected to the power of intention, everywhere you go, and everyone you meet, is affected by you and the energy you radiate. As you become the power of intention, you'll see your dreams being fulfilled almost magically, and you'll see yourself creating huge ripples in the energy fields of others by your presence and nothing more...

...When you shift to an abundance mind-set, you repeat to yourself over and over again that you're unlimited because you emanated from the inexhaustible supply of intention. As this picture solidifies, you begin to act on this attitude of unbending intent. There's no other possibility...

– *Wayne W. Dyer, The Power of Intention: Learning to Co-create Your World Your Way*

9. Heal

With healing intentions clear and with focus on healing, ask for help from your spirit team, tell them you love them, thank them for being there and thank them for the healing that is taking place. This is part of the grounding process before you begin performing further healing actions. It is important for each person to find that place where they feel connected. Some do it through visualizing themselves as a tree with roots dug deep into the earth and branches connected to heaven. Some pray.

During this grounding process, spend some time in mediation and/or prayer. Look at an object, pay attention to your breathing and bring your mind to the present moment. Acknowledging any emotions that need to be recognized, felt and resolved. Move them to a mental to do list, for later if needed. Acknowledge specific things that you are grateful for. Request help to forgive (if needed). Let go of any obstacles though acceptance and forgiveness. Focus compassion on the person in need. Then while feeling compassion and gratitude, focus on the detailed intention using visualizations. In your mind see the end result and see the healing as having already happened. Then when ready, move into Visionwork or Thetawork healing as follows:

VISIONWORK: In your mind, form a detailed anatomically correct 3D vision of the person in need and their ailment. Communicate with the cells and watch them respond to your energy and the energy around them. Watch this image for an extended period of time as lights, or water, or energy sparks, nibbles away at the diseased area, dissolving it to the point of being replaced by healthy tissue and function. Continue to hold the connection to your heart as you do this. Keep focused over as long a period of time as you can hold, watching the healing unfold in your mind's eye.

THETAWORK: Theta is the first stage of the phase when we dream. To understand this frequency in a simple and comprehensive enough to think about how it feels and what it's like being on top of a mountain totally absorbed by what's around you, knowing that you "know" (not just believe) that your higher power, the source or creator, is real and just "is". Breathe deeply and take yourself to the point before you fall asleep into lucid dreaming. At that moment you are in Theta, a deeply relaxed and dream-like state.

Then with your consciousness, perceive yourself leaving your body. As energy, visualize moving upward past the earth's stratosphere, through the layer of all knowledge where past-present-future are all one. Then move up into the light, thank your higher power, the source or creator, for the healing having already happened. Then, as energy, travel back down into the person in need and with brilliant light, bring vitality to the areas in need of healing. Watch as everything becomes corrected and purified. Then take your spirit energy back up to the light in gratitude and then back down into your body.

Then pair up with your partner if in groups. As the healer, sit or stand with feet firmly planted like roots. Imagine you being connected to the energy of heaven and the earth below. While feeling compassion and gratitude, connect to spirit, open your heart. Then complete the healing task with Reiki or Therapeutic Touch® (TT). In The Code, healing is finalized with TT as follows:

Therapeutic Touch® (TT): TT was first brought to our attention in 1972 as a modern healing method, by Dolores Krieger, PhD, RN, and her colleague, Dora Kunz. Together, they standardized a technique that has been referred to as a contemporary interpretation of several ancient healing practices. TT is a holistic, evidence-based therapy that incorporates the intentional and compassionate use of universal energy to promote balance and well-being. It is a consciously-directed process during which the practitioner uses the hands as a focus to facilitate the healing process. The intent is to re-pattern the client's energy field toward wholeness and health thereby enhancing their own ability to heal.

TT can be compared to Reiki in that the hands are placed over the person's body sensing the energy field and noting anomalies in it. The field communicates with the person facilitating the healing. Disruptions in the field can be felt as temperature changes, spikes, excess that is not congruent with patterns in the rest of the body. Then the healing facilitator moves the hands and creates visualizations to smooth out or balance these irregularities.

In TT often the therapist does not know what the detailed issues are. They do not have a detailed statement of intention but rely on the energy field itself to inform the practitioner. Here in this Code for Empowered Healing, we deviate by also keeping the intentions in mind as we use our hands to facilitate those intentions. Here however, one must always trust the field and the signals it is communicating above the man-made intentions created and treat the person as they are, with what is found. The following is not the official version of how TT is done, please see a teacher certified in TT for classes. This what is done for The Code:

Perform TT once grounded. Ask the person for permission and tell them what you are planning to do. Move the hands over the body's energy field approximately 6 inches away. This will depend of where you feel the edge of the field. Note the qualities and symmetry of what you sense. If any areas feel out of balance, go back again over the body and in your mind visualize heat, or colours or move the hands to smooth out any anomalies. Go back over the body as often as needed until the field feels more balanced. Then touch the person's feet to ground their energy when finished and ask how they are doing.

Close Circle

If there is a group, everyone should wait quietly until everyone has completed healing and being healed. Then have everyone come back to the circle. You should remain inside the sacred space until the circle is closed. Have everyone close their eyes and visualize the energy flowing in the opposite direction of the earth's rotation from east to west to undo the circle. Speak aloud and offer gratitude for the source of all life, your spirit allies and all those that attended. Then ask for or read a blessing** aloud before anyone leaves the circle.

**Blessing:*

*We were created to be healthy & happy.
Like the earth we undergo
a cycle of transformation
That is beautiful and perfect.
Awaken to this rebirth and be in awe
of the magic of each moment.
Feel the peace of gratitude envelop you.
See your true self in the reflection
of the still waters of your soul.
Know that you are perfect just as you are,
wonderfully made and worthy of love.
Specially created and unique.
Accept the care and respect and know you are
deserving of your rightful place.
-SG Williams*

Final Notes on Methods

You can modify these healing methods by choosing techniques you are already familiar with. Please alter the spiritual meditations, blessings and rituals for creating a circle, to those that fit with your own beliefs and preferences. These methods can be used alone or in a group. If you are alone, you can do this for yourself or someone else. When alone, keeping your healing circle members in mind and honouring their healing intentions, after the session when you are doing this for yourself, adds to the power of compassion for your own healing.

You can meet as a Healing Group often as you like and/or splinter off and form new groups. Each group will develop its own ground rules and practices. It is important that what happens and what is said in the group, must stay in the group. Healing circles should be a safe place for all who enter. Once you see how to raise the vibration of the group, each person can continue with their own version of *The Code for Empowered Healing* practice. That is the hope.

8 THE CODE

Some of the techniques I used came to me in a dream and I have yet to be able to explain all the reasons why I choose to do things this way. For example each of the 9 activities in the method, is done in either 3, 6 or 9 repetitions. The diagram I created to visually portray The diagram for *The Code for Empowered Healing*, at the end of this chapter (and on the cover), is drawn with these numbers.

In ancient times numbers often had spiritual meanings. Numerology is a sacred holistic art that studies the meaning of numbers and their patterns, even in modern times. The number 3, represents the emerging awareness of the divine aspects of the mind, body and spiritual unity. The number 6, taps into our imagination and the power that creativity invokes. The number 9, allows us to enter through the doorway of creation, into our true, higher self, as we awaken to the connected-ness and oneness of universal consciousness.

Vortex Math studies the patterns of numbers and their qualities, not just quantities. Some consider this pseudo-science a pile of bunk. It is however widely known and popularized. In this practice the polarizing numbers 1, 2, 4, 5, 7 and 8 represent the material world. Number 3, 6, and 9 govern the physical and represent the non-material unseen spiritual world. Number 9 appears most frequently when the measure of the sides of shapes are summed or when measuring the circumference of a circle. All measures in the natural world reduce to the numbers 3, 6 or 9. For example all notes in the Solfeggio harmonic scale of 432 Hz add up to 3, 6 or 9 and all snowflakes and the shapes of a bee's honeycomb are six sided.

Tesla thought these numbers were the fundamental language of the universe. He thought 3 was for energy, 6 for vibration and 9 for frequency. Because he believed we are energetically one with everything around us, Tesla's 369 code combined thought, feelings and beliefs as vibrational frequencies that shape our universe at all levels from the unseen to the physical according to the unified field theory. Now it is popular for people to use 369 in methods for manifesting their desires.

If only you knew the magnificence of the 3, 6 and 9, then you would have the key to the universe -
Nikola Tesla

The Code Sequence – Condensed Overview

---------A – Prepare---------

a) Gather your people with the intention to clear and purify the space of negative energy and emotions.

b) Use tuning forks, incense, essential oils, or sweet grass or other herbs. People can smudge themselves with sacred smoke if desired.

c) Then you can use sounds to raise the vibrations. Use drums and drumming, tuning forks, singing bowls, gongs, healing music, chanting or toning, for as long as you like.

---------B - Open Circle---------

(a) Have everyone close their eyes and visualize the energy flowing in the direction of the earth's rotation (west to east).

(b) Speak aloud that "only love may enter this circle". Clear your thoughts, become present and allow all negativity to drift away.

(c) Ask aloud for a blessing from the source of all life and for the support of spirit allies (use your own belief system here).

---------C - Perform 9 Healing Activities---------

I – Body - Qi

1. <u>Increase Qi</u>: Increase and awaken the physical energy of your body using Qigong exercises of the Eight Brocade. You can use other techniques you may know such as Tai Chi or Yoga. Do repetitions of each of the 9 moves.

2. <u>Activate Meridians</u>: Tune the body and increase energy flow by tapping the meridians and acupressure points on a few specific points of your choice on the main meridians. Do in repetitions of 6 taps for each of the 6 sets of points.

3. <u>Direct Qi</u>: Do some visualization and hand positioning over the 3 main energy centres to activate and increase the energy resources of the body. Do 9 repetitions for the set of 3 energy centres.

II – Mind- Energy

4. <u>Calm Mind</u>: Do some deep breathing and toning with vocalized sounds for each energy area (Weng, Ar, Hong) at the same time using the energy ball visualization and then say, "Thank you" 3 times, for the 3 beings (your body, your spirit allies, your higher power), for each of the 3 energy centres.

5. <u>Clear Thoughts</u>: Spend time in quiet, silent personal meditation and/or prayer. Pay

attention to your breathing and bring your mind to the present moment. Allow thoughts to wander in and out acknowledging any emotions that need to be recognized. Let go of any obstacles. Spend 6 minutes in meditation.

6. Direct Mind: Have someone read positive affirmations (such as I am loved, I am worthy, I am healed) or create your own silently, to seed the mind with positive thoughts. Repeat these 9 times.

III – Spirit - Soul

7. Set Intention: Gather the knowledge you need for the healing task required using the details you know about specific ailments with detailed biological information. Some members may share with the group such details as desired. Repeat the intention 6 times to yourself.

8. Open Heart: Read a specific scripted Heart Meditation* aloud to expand compassion and open the heart. Pick 3 people to focus on for your love and compassion.

9. Heal: In your mind see the end result and see the healing as having already happened using Visionwork or Thetawork. Split off with your partner and perform healing actions by clearing negative thoughts, centring, grounding and focusing on the healing required. Then execute healing actions using acupressure, Reiki and/or Therapeutic

Touch® to expand on that healing. Do the healing for a minimum of 9 minutes on each person. Then switch roles. Remain quiet until everyone is finished.

---------D - Close Circle---------

(a) Come back to the circle. Have everyone close their eyes and visualize the energy flowing east to west.

(b) Speak aloud and offer gratitude for the source of all life, your spirit allies and all those that attended.

(c) Then ask for or read a blessing** aloud before anyone leaves the circle.

The Code Diagram

The diagram of the Code (next page) shows a star where the 3 figures intersect in the middle. This is the portal to connectivity with the universal spirit or higher power. Using the Code to harness the power of healing is cyclical, as we spin up into higher realms and higher frequencies in our 9 exercises, we create a vortex through which we can enter the intersecting portal to be connected with the Creator. We might be more successful in some sessions in others as we are trying to achieve a perfect storm. However the strength of love, our compassion and our intentions are the main factors that bring about successful healing.

The Code for Empowered Healing

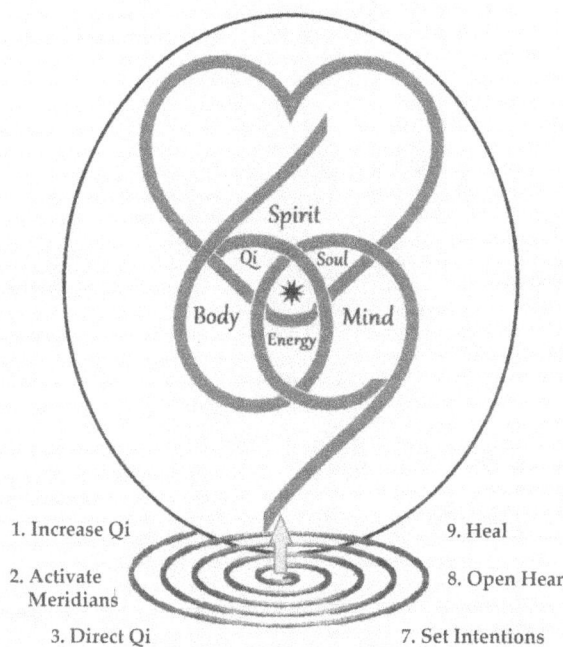

1. Increase Qi
2. Activate Meridians
3. Direct Qi
4. Calm Mind
5. Clear Thoughts
6. Direct Mind
7. Set Intentions
8. Open Heart
9. Heal

FOUNDATION

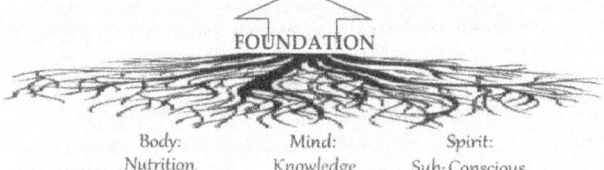

Body:	Mind:	Spirit:
Nutrition	Knowledge	Sub-Conscious
Movement	Introspection	Soul Self
Surroundings	Consciousness	Love

9 Mastery and Transcendence

The Power of Being

"When you want something, all the universe conspires in helping you to achieve it."
– Paulo Coelho

We are all healers if we want to be. The more solid our foundation, the more we will be able to heal because this feeds the quality and quantity of energy we can harness. If we seek to continue the path of a healer, we can achieve mastery and transcendence that will allow us to resonate with the world around us. In this we can experience true peace no matter what happens to us, or around us. In everything we can find an abundance of joy and love by just being our true selves.

In those moments when we are in nature, or feel a deep connection with the universe, we often feel joyous, elated, thankful and a sense of wonder. If we learn how to tap into these frequencies, or synchronize with these vibrations, on a regular basis, we can find in us, a source of creativity and passion. This place where we find the source, or access it within ourselves, transforms us. This is a place where we begin to learn that we are loved, just the way we are.

However this is not a reality for most of us who struggle with being human. What most of us do feel, is that the ego is like a mask we wear at a masquerade party called life. That is why we need to take trips to "find ourselves" or "get away from ourselves" for a while. What are we getting away from? It is the actor in the play, we are tired of playing. We know there is more to the world and ourselves. That is why philosophers, religions and psychologists, do what they do. It is why so many are depressed, looking for a reason to be on this earth. However, the religious stories, musings of philosophers and the drugs, are not working. Who we are, needs to make sense to us and we need to know what is really going on.

Being able to maneuver through the world without being bullied by our subconscious nature and our demanding ego, is a skill that we practice from birth. We are all ducks floating along gracefully on the surface of society, while our legs are paddling like mad beneath the surface, just so we can appear normal and fit in. We all suffer the internal wars between what we know we should do, what we really want to do and what we are driven to do. The heart longs for freedom, while our minds keep warning us of the dangers. Our heart says it has the key, but our mind keeps us in cages, even after the locks have been opened.

We all face fear, doubt, strife and drama. We are always looking for more, to be better, to be loved and most of all, to be free. But who is running our lives? Are we living our lives or are we just reacting to what life throws at us? People try to do better, find God, religion, happiness, or the right partner, hoping to find the magic IT. The real miracle is that you don't have to be better, find God, religion, a partner, or be in the right circumstances to find bliss and freedom. The gift is free, if you stop listening to the ego, let go of being controlled by the mind and let the higher you, real you, find its centre and its voice.

The reality is that you cannot, in all honesty, be better than you already are. Our good and bad, yin and yang are all amazingly wonderful, awesome beyond belief. Even the angels are envious of us. Tuning into the higher frequency channel, allows you to see your greatness and that there is nothing to fear. Neither death nor life are any better than the other. You have always been and always will be you. Everything you need to be happy is there for the taking, anytime. You are a powerful being, you matter and the universe cares for us, but we just don't know it. Are you not much more valuable than these?:

Look at the birds of the air, they do not sow or reap or store away in barns, and yet your heavenly Father feeds them. - Matthew 6:26

...

> *...The great Tao flows unobstructed in every direction. All things rely on it to conceive and be born, and it does not deny even the smallest of creatures... Lao Tzu, the Tao Te Ching*

We are loved despite the imperfections that are a mirror of everything that exists in the universe. We see that our multifaceted nature of good and evil, brave and cowardly, selfish and generous, kind and mean, honest and deceitful ways, are what it means to be human. We are healed and made whole as we learn it is OK to be human. The omnipresent creator made us and accepts us just the way we are. Over time, we come to realize how much unconditional love comes our way.

The key is living in the moment. Not thinking about the past and carrying old baggage into the now. It is not about a constant preoccupation with our plans and possible future events. Worry about the future is a constant drag on the journey. To just say stop, to living in the past, or the future, is asking us to do something that is next to impossible for most of us. Your greatest power lies in this very present moment because this is when you can actually do something that creates ripples into tomorrow and the future.

Through our passions and creativity, we are co-creators with the divine source. Eventually, the "real" you can take charge of the ego and mind chatter. The way in which we direct our power, once obtained, is through our thoughts, intentions, visualization and our hands.

Where you put your hands, is where energy goes...Where you focus your mind is where you boost energy and heal...To meld with Tao is to reach immortality... - Tao I (The Way of All Life) by Master Zhi Gang Sha

I call it "being in the zone" and liken it to surfing high on the crest of a wave, above the din of human drama, where the view is splendid, the air vibrant and fresh. On this wave, one is filled with intense expectancy, where one has to keep focused and balanced to keep from falling into the sea. From this vantage point, what you visualize, sing, chant, focus on and are grateful for receiving, as if it has already happened, will come to fruition.

...whatever you have asked for in prayer, believe that you have received it, and it will be yours... - Mark 11:24

Acceptance of the greatness, of who we really are, comes with the ability to see the world like a child again, with magic and wonder behind everyday events. Knowing your true self, gives you the freedom from judging yourself and others and a new perspective, as to why you are here. Not only is this liberating, but spending time in your soul of eternity, takes you into a certain vibration and resonance with a world, freer from conflict, more at peace, filled with more love. This is the power of being.

The Power of Connection

If we are the expression of and the extended frequencies of the higher power, what do we know and believe about that? Religions with man made rules no longer make sense for everyone. It is not logical that a loving God allows bad things to happen. Eastern religions, philosophy and psychology are foreign to many of us in the west. Living an austere life under strict rules in a monk-hood does not sit well with those of us who want to find our own way. In just the same way the monasteries and lives lived by some of the more well known Christian saints, do not make sense either. The cornucopia of gurus from every walk of life, confuse us with their messages and drown out our own experiential knowing.

Each of us must pick our way through all the stories and find what makes sense for us. We are not capable of seeing the complete picture, with our human brains, anyway. We need to rely on the communication of ideas, with words, that will always over simplify and taint the real truth. However we can know and recognize truth in the messages of the vibrations we feel when we resonate with them. We have a sense of knowing what rings true for us.

Experiments in Quantum Physics have shown how a molecule is able to spontaneously change back and forth between being a wave and a particle. How you ("the observer") choose to perceive the particle influences this behaviour. What is interesting about these experiments, is that the simple act of observing the experiment influences the results. It shows that we are not separate from the smallest of atoms.

Everything is connected.

Our ego operates at a different wavelength and tends to reside in our mind, or at least is reinforced with our mind. In order to act within the guideposts considered normal in society, it takes a fair amount of negotiation and harmony between the three aspects of animal nature, the ego and our higher self. How we move through life depends on our successes in the way we manage these.

It is in our synchronicity with the divine that we find power. It is not our own personal power as such. It is the power of the universe that we accept and allow to flow through us, once we know how to live in a way that we can connect to it. It is the unifying power of all the universe that we are trusted to wield in our unity with it. Practicing our connection to the highest frequencies of our creator, gives us the ability to step away from the internal battles and see what is real.

> *The masters of old attained unity with the Tao...*
> *Humanity attained unity so that they might*
> *flourish...This is the power of unity... - Lao Tzu*

Eventually you can access your power as it flows through you as an extension of God, the goddess, the higher power, Tao, or Brahman, as your true self learns to resonate with this. This harmonious synchronicity is how we receive and understand the vibrational signals. Over time, that still small voice, as Elijah described the way in which God spoke to him, will become stronger in us. There are many ways in which we can build that relationship with our true self. The power is in just "Being" and flowing with the present moment. According to the Tao, this kind of connection with God, the Divine or Tao includes a number of steps:

- First, remove all sickness (healing the self physically, emotionally, mentally and spiritually);

- Secondly, go (beyond healing) to transform old age to that of a baby (reclaiming youth);

- Then finally, reaching the state of human, Mother Earth, Heaven or Tao sainthood. Where sainthood is equated with being the servant. A Tao saint achieves immortality, where healing of the soul comes before physical healing and where healing of all the universes requires balancing and harmonizing at all levels to the frequency of Tao.

Saints who melded with Tao since ancient time, completely connected and melded with Heaven and Earth. They mastered yin and yang. They breathed and received nourishment from the essence of the universe.

...

Concentrate and focus on your soul, heart and mind. Use your mind to focus inside your body. Meld soul, heart, mind and body as one. Life is as long as Heaven's and Earth's. Physical life has no ending.
  − Chapter 1 of the Important Wisdom of Tao

The God frequency allows us to vibrate at the highest emotions of love, compassion and joy. The work of trying to be good is no longer necessary. Just as you are loved, you will love others and all motives, in everything you do, will flow from that good place. As Saint Augustine is quoted as saying, "Love and do what you will". The resonating connection gives you the courage you need to take risks, be creative and live to the fullest of abandonment that you choose. You have the power of the universe at your fingertips and you can create the world of your dreams in every present moment. It doesn't matter if you go through hell, you will still be free and filled with joy even in the darkest of places. This is the power of connection.

Supercharged Intention

One of the first things I learned at acupuncture school was to set my intention at the tip of the needle. What does that mean? I knew it was an important lesson, but it would be years before I realized just what that meant. Whole books have been written about how important intention is. Then as I learned Therapeutic Touch®, I experienced how intention combined with compassion was a key ingredient for healing.

I have read from Wayne Dyer, that if you are connected to the power of intention, you radiate energy that affects everyone around you, like ripples in a pond. When you see that your intention brings about your desires, your belief in its abundance grows and creates a fountain of power. You start to manifest your world by co-creating it with intention.

Staying focused on a detailed intention can be difficult. Many healers have fine tuned this to an art and have taught many people how to do this. In Theta Healing, visualization helps you watch the healing take place as you thank the universe that the healing is done. The key here is that you ask and see that it is fulfilled, right there and then. No hoping for it to happen in the future. It is done.

The intention of a healer is to always help, not harm. Always to be open and caring. Intention is powerful. It is more than that however. After a decade of using my skills to help people heal, I found that compassion is equally as important. A mentor I highly respect, Dr. Franklin Chen, told a class of graduating acupuncturists, *"The most important thing you can do is to love your patients. They will know if you love them or not"*.

Love is actioned through compassion. You can't really help people heal, if you are not compassionate. You can't be compassionate if you don't love. You can't love them if you judge them and don't see them as they really are. I had the privilege of hearing the stories of struggle, triumph and defeat and seeing strength and beauty in each client. I was often in awe and I believe this is a reflection of how the angels see us.

We are all heroes, heroines and warriors, each in his and her own right. As my husband says, we are all the number one stars in our own life. If you do really listen, and see others, the dynamics of healer and patient together, opens up a shared energy field. Here is where spirit allies come in and commune with you. It is a powerful experience where high level frequencies are supercharged. Each person comes away with new insights and inspiration.

To be in balance everyday and not take on the woes of your patients, takes a dedicated spiritual practice. Some call it grounding but however you do it, you need to connect to the earth's energy, the spirit within you and the omnipresent spirit that surrounds you. If you don't, you can get pulled into the emotions and drama of your clients, creating an imbalance. This will exhaust you of your own limited resources. However connecting to the source, by practising the art of gratitude every day (as one way), provides the endless energy and passion needed. This becomes easier over time. It also makes life so much more enjoyable when you see the world through a thankful window.

It is in that mix, that a healer experiences intention fuelled by compassion, supported by spirit, through the gateway of gratitude. This is really a three legged stool that supports our words and the detailed vision of what we want to create for ourselves and others. When you add prayer, which I do, this is the stuff of miracles. The result of this combination based in love, creates a high frequency healing bubble filled with, what I call, supercharged intention.

In the universe there is an immeasurable, indescribable force which shamans call intent, and absolutely everything that exists in the entire cosmos is attached to intent by a connecting link. - Carlos Castaneda

...

The power of intention is the power to manifest, to create, to live a life of unlimited abundance, and to attract into your life the right people at the right moments. - Wayne Dyer

...

The highest intention comes from love and compassion ... when our intentions come from a place of love and compassion then we have the power of the universe... Intentions compressed into words enfold magical power.- Deepak Chopra

The Magic of Resonance

Resonance is about the vibes in us, those we were born with and those we cultivate through our physical and mental health. It is about the vibes in the environment that surrounds us and those relationships that support us. It is about how all these vibes "sync-up", balance and resonate with all the other vibes flowing through our reality. Our self-organized vibrational fields and complex resonance of these frequencies, make up our consciousness. Scientists studying the Resonance Theory of Consciousness, say "shared resonance through specific neuron electrochemical firing patterns creates an electromagnetic field that may itself be the seat of macro-consciousness".

Our sense of self therefore, comes from the harmonious vibrations that we feel as the seer behind our eyes. This can happen when we quiet ourselves and become aware of the music of ourselves, as a small still voice in our hearts. This spontaneous self-organization of the expression of our DNA blueprint of millions of oscillating fields, is our perception that "I am Me". As we awaken, it becomes apparent that the key to knowing ourselves lies in the synchronicity with the universal high frequency energies in everything. We are not just a Me.

Quantum Entanglement in physics describes how a group of particles become acquainted by interacting together in the same space. They become indistinguishable appearing as one entity in a quantum state. Then when the particles are separated, even over long distances, they still cannot be distinguished independently from the whole. Even at long distances, the particles will recognize one another as part of themselves. We too are more than our individual cells when we resonate and therefore tap into a collective power of creation. We recognize those things that resonate with us, even if we can't see them.

We are part of an "Us" who is integral to the shared consciousness of God, Spirit, Tao, Brahman or higher power. We have always been associated with that same energy that created us in the first place, inseparable as in a quantum state. Therefore it is up to us to accept this wonderful insight and use our power wisely by "living correctly", in harmony with the seasons and all the earth's inhabitants.

Find Your Tribe

Believe it or not there are people out there just like you. No matter how weird you think you or your beliefs are. You are not alone and when you think you are, the universe will send someone to walk along your path with you, even if for just a little while. Some of us go through life thinking we were either born into the wrong family, born in the wrong century or for some, we think we may have landed on the wrong planet.

It takes time to learn what a good relationship looks like. Some of us are lucky enough to see it first hand with role models. Most of us learn by trial and error as we experience what it feels like, to be around people that help us feel at peace with ourselves or not. We feel at peace when we are accepted for who we are by both others and ourselves.

Even better is to find someone who is interested in us and cares enough to actually listen and hear what we are saying. These valuable friends want to know the real you, not make assumptions about who they think you are. Often you can feel a connection with the people who get-you. You are not a role in a play on the stage, planet earth. Don't be afraid to venture out beyond your known circle if you find yourself stuck with the wrong friends.

Good friends are those you can trust with your feelings and who are willing to reciprocate. They are the folks you can go to when times are difficult and feel safe. They are the folks that will not abandon you when you make mistakes or have a difference of opinion. Even if you can find one such person with whom you can experience just some of these attributes, this is priceless.

That resonance of energy with like minded folks gives you a sense of belonging and that you matter. Good relationships help you to see yourself in a better light through the eyes of those who love you and respect you. You can feel with your heart energy, who and what is right for you, when you practice paying attention to it. Your tribe will help you increase your energy and accelerate your own healing.

Healing takes love, compassion, intention, divine help and friends. Some of us have spent a major part of our lives searching for this. Don't stop. This world needs healing right now. There are lots of folks out there, with the stuff needed to make that happen. I know because I have been privileged to meet so many of them, in my healing practice. There are many good souls out there, being that pebble that is spreading ripples of healing energy out to the world.

In a nutshell however, the fundamentals are that to heal others and heal the world, we need to be on a healing journey for ourselves. Learning who we really are and the power of just being, is where we tap into that oneness with everything and everyone else. As we become whole and experience the power of connection, we are able to transcend the human condition of struggle. In this state we have no choice but to magically resonate with the qualities and properties of the source, which is love. That love moves us to compassion where we want to help ease the suffering of others. We are compelled to master our skills and fine tune our intentions, to help others. Therefore seek to heal and be healed and in the process you will heal the world. I believe there is no greater purpose than this.

Living with Purpose

It is our purpose and destiny to live in conscious oneness with our world, be present and know that our true identity is in the reflection of the divine.

...

When your non-persona can tap into your passion and your actions are directed by love, inspiration and enthusiasm, your work will resonate in alignment with the goals of the universe.

...

This is the secret to knowing your life purpose. A purpose that you can fulfill every day, you have the courage to be true to what you know and what is right.

...

In this way, you will change the world, with more power than any one person could ever imagine or accomplish.

- SG Williams

ABOUT THE AUTHOR

SG Williams is a holistic health specialist with a background in traditional Chinese medicine, acupuncture, herbology and Therapeutic Touch®, as well as science research. For over more than three decades she has been involved in healthcare in some way. In the last decade she has successfully operated her own healing clinic, treating a wide range of complex issues encompassing mental, emotional, spiritual and physical well-being. Her ultimate goal for her patients was not just restored health, but to see them able to be in the world, as their true selves. She believes that this is what true healing is all about.

www.ingramcontent.com/pod-product-compliance
Lightning Source LLC
Chambersburg PA
CBHW061956070426
42450CB00011BA/3049